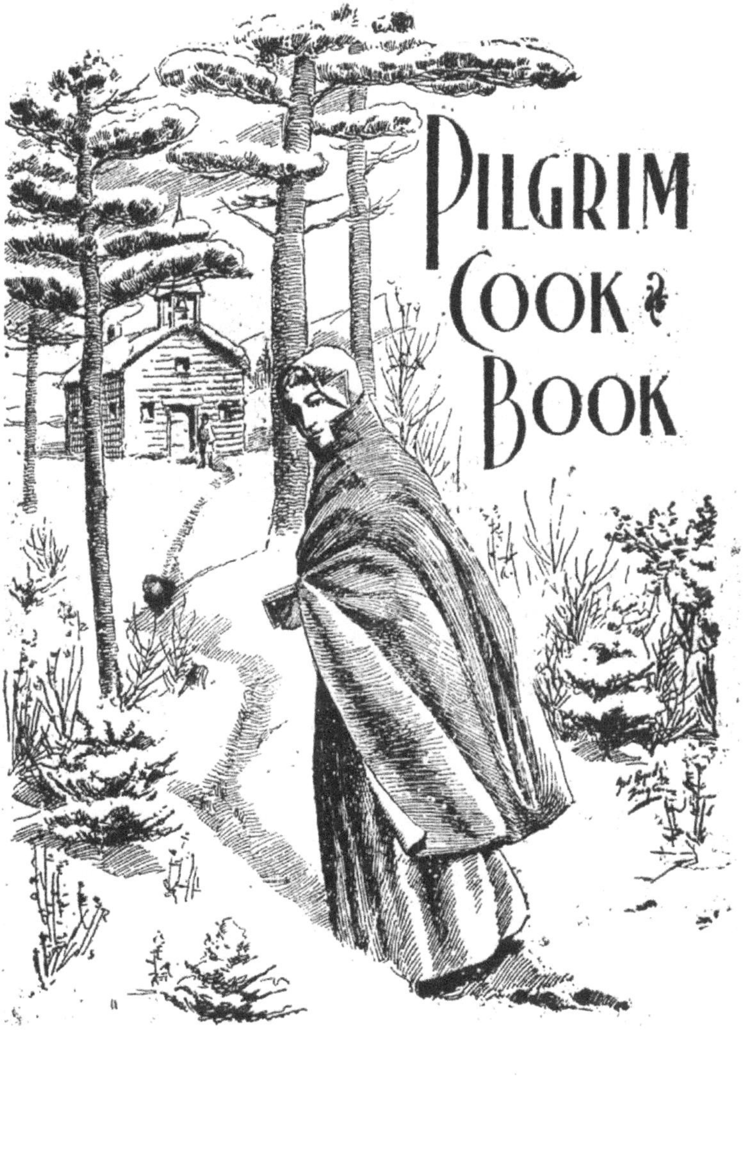
Pilgrim
Cook
Book

Presented to
Michigan State College
by
Mr & Mrs Thos. Gunson

June 1940

The Pilgrim Cook Book.

No home can be what it ought to be unless there is a good cook in the establishment.—Mrs. Emma P. Ewing.

COMPILED BY THE LADIES OF

Pilgrim Congregational Church

LANSING, MICHIGAN

1895

Darius D. Thorp & Son, Printers and Binders
Lansing, Michigan

Our Greeting.

TO ALL WOMEN who live to learn and would learn to live, these pages are offered by the compilers, in the hope that they may prove crumbs of comfort in many perplexing hours. We desire to thank all kind contributors and all who have added anything to the success of our undertaking. Careful attention to details, we believe, will prove every recipe offered to be valuable. We especially invite attention to the "Diet for the Sick," prepared by one of national fame for this little book. In the abundance of material offered, lack of space compelled the omission of many gond things. In a few instances, the recipes sent by kind friends were unsigned, so that due credit could not be given.

WE HAVE
FOR THE
HOLIDAYS

New Bibles, Testaments, Prayer and Hymnals, Gift Books, Art Books, the Poets and Standard Authors,

GOLD PENS, OPERA GLASSES, POCKET BOOKS, LETTER TABLETS, ALBUMS, TOILET SETS, CHILDREN'S BOOKS, GAMES, ETC.

AGENTS FOR THE WATERMAN FOUNTAIN PEN.

18 DIARIES 96

CROTTY BROTHERS,

206 WASHINGTON AVE. NORTH.

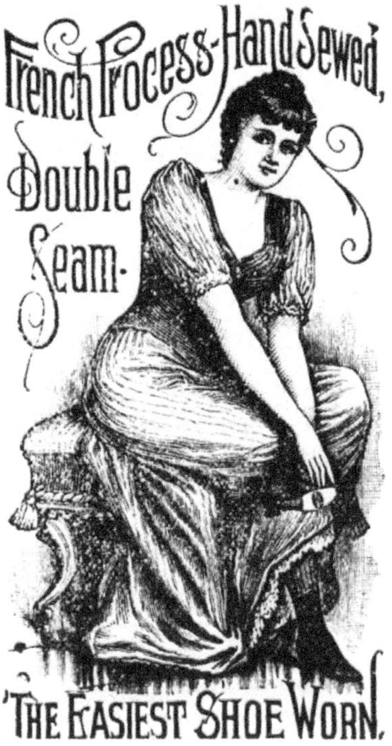

THE

"New Woman"

Requires shoes that are strictly "up to date," and the . . .

New "Tokio"

is the latest, easiest, and most practical of the new styles. . .

Fine Dongola Kid, light soles, lace or button	$3 00
Box Calf, for wet weather, extension soles	3 75
Vici Kid, lace or button, extension soles	3 50
French Enamel, waterproof, heavy extension soles	5 00
Finest Paris Kid, turned soles, very light and dainty	5 00
Patent Leather, same style as last	5 00

...YOURS TRULY...

G. D. WOODBURY,

103 WASHINGTON AVENUE SOUTH.

Soups.

"The kitchen is a laboratory where the record of experiment is kept, not in note-books, but in the health and spirits of the family."

Bouillon.—To three pounds of raw meat, chopped fine, add three quarts of cold water; let it barely warm for the first hour, then increase the heat and let it gently simmer for six hours, stirring it occasionally; turn it into an earthen vessel; salt to taste and cover till cool; skim off all the fat, squeeze the meat hard as you remove it from the liquid, throw in the shell and white of a raw egg, put the liquor over the fire in a clean saucepan, bring it quickly to a boiling point, boil rapidly ten minutes; each quart of water put to the raw beef should have simmered down to a pint, then strain carefully through a cloth. Do not squeeze it as it should be a clear amber color. Bouillon for lunches or other entertainments, should be served very hot and no spoons. For family use either hot or cold as preferred.

Bean Soup.—Soak over night one pint of beans in three pints of water. In the morning drain, add fresh water. Set over fire; remove the skins as much as possible as they come to the top; boil until perfectly soft; add flour and butter rubbed together and season with pepper and salt.

Cream of Celery Soup.—One pint of milk, a tablespoonful of flour, one of butter, a head of celery, a large slice of onion, and a small piece of mace. Boil celery after cutting into inch pieces or smaller, from thirty to forty minutes, boil mace, onion and milk together. Mix flour with two tablespoonfuls of cold milk and add to boiling milk. Cook ten minutes. Wash celery in the water in which it has been cooked and stir into boiling milk. Add butter, season with salt and pepper to taste. Strain and serve immediately. —*Mrs. F. L. Dodge.*

BEEF STOCK.—Take a shank of beef, wash thoroughly, cut in pieces and crack the bones, cover with four quarts of water, let come to a boil quickly, skim and then boil slowly until the water is half boiled away, remove meat, strain and salt to taste.

TOMATO SOUP, No. 1.—Take pieces of roast beef and beefsteak that are left from dinner and breakfast, and boil till the juice is extracted; to one quart of liquor add a quart of stewed tomatoes, boil and strain, season with salt and pepper and serve hot.

TOMATO SOUP, No. 2.—To one pint of canned tomatoes or four large ones, cut fine, add one quart of boiling water and let them boil; then add one teaspoon of soda, when it will foam. Immediately add one pint of sweet milk with salt, pepper and plenty of butter. When this boils add a little rolled cracker and serve. Equal to oyster soup.

GREEN CORN SOUP.—Twelve ears tender corn cut from cobs; boil the cobs twenty minutes in two quarts of water, remove cobs, boil the corn twenty minutes, add one quart of milk, season with pepper, salt and butter to taste, then turn into a tureen in which the yolks of three eggs have been beaten.

ENGLISH SOUP.—Take any kind of meat for stock—beef, mutton, or veal or gravies. Put in your kettle with about one quart of water. When it boils nicely put in a little of every kind of vegetable you have and a small handful of rolled oats; season with salt and pepper and a little tomato. If you use soup bone let it boil about two hours before you put in the vegetables; take out the meat, cut a few pieces off the bone and put in the kettle again. The cabbage and onion leaves an unpleasant flavor in the meat when it is cold. What meat is left is nice to use for hash or meat pie.

Mock Bisque Soup.—One can of tomatoes. While they are stewing put three pints of milk on to boil. When it boils stir in one heaping tablespoon of flour which has been mixed with a little cold milk. Let them boil ten minutes. Then add butter size of a small egg, and salt and pepper to taste. Strain tomatoes and add one teaspoon of soda and stir in the milk. Serve immediately.—*Mrs. W. S. Griswold.*

Bean Soup.—One pint of beans washed and cooked until partly done; add ¼ teaspoonful of soda and stir thoroughly through the beans. Drain off this water and add more boiling water, cook until perfectly done. Rub through colander and season with salt, pepper and butter. Thin with milk and heat again before serving.—*Mrs. George Pratt.*

Potato Soup.—One quart of milk, six large potatoes, one stalk celery, one onion, one tablespoon butter; put milk to boil with onion and celery; pare potatoes, boil thirty minutes, mash fine and light, add boiling milk, butter, salt and pepper to taste. A cup of whipped cream added is excellent.

Potato Soup.—A delicious soup, easily and quickly made.

Take four good sized potatoes, pare, boil and mash them smoothly, have ready two quarts of sweet milk in which three stalks of celery have been put heated to nearly boiling, taking care not to scorch the milk. Take out the celery and stir in the potatoes, stirring well till it comes to a boil. Whip to a froth four tablespoonfuls of good sweet cream and stir into it after it is ready for the table. It should be served immediately after the cream is stirred in. Season to taste.—*Mrs. O. M. Barnes.*

VERMICELLI SOUP.—To make vermicelli soup, take as much good stock as you require for your tureen, strain, and set it on the fire, and when it boils put in the vermicelli. Let it simmer for half an hour by a slow fire that the vermicelli may not break. The soup ought not to be very thick. Half a pound of vermicelli is sufficient for eight or ten persons.

POTATO SOUP.—To each quart of soup required, boil a pint of sliced potatoes and a slice or two of white onion in enough water to cover them. When done add a pint of rich milk, a little salt; let come to a boil, add a teaspoon flour rubbed smooth with a little milk and a piece of butter. Let come to a boil and serve.—*Mrs. Geo. Ritter.*

CONSOMME.—Try out two thin slices of bacon, and brown one sliced onion in the dripping. Take two pounds of lean beef and two pounds of veal, cut in small pieces, add the onion, and brown slightly. Cover with four quarts of cold water and simmer for four hours. Add two sprigs of parsley, one stalk of celery, half of a small carrot, and a small piece of lemon peel. Simmer one hour longer, strain through a sieve, and stand away to cool. When cold remove the fat from the surface, clarify, and when ready to use color with caramel.—*Saginaw Cook Book.*

CREAM OF ASPARAGUS SOUP.—Cut off, about an inch in length, the points of two bunches of asparagus, and simmer them gently until tender in water sufficient to cover them, to which a teaspoonful of salt has been added. Boil the stalks of the asparagus twenty minutes in three pints of soup stock, or water, then strain and thicken the liquid with a tablespoonful of flour, let it boil two minutes, and add a pint of sweet cream and the asparagus points with the water in which they were cooked. Season with salt and pepper and serve hot.—*Mrs. Emma P. Ewing.*

CROUTONS—Or fried bread crumbs for soups, are prepared in this way: Cut slices of stale home made bread half an inch thick, trim off all crust, and cut each slice into squares; fry these in very hot fat; drain them on a clean napkin, or brown paper, and add six or eight to each portion of soup.

FISH AND SHELL FISH.

FRIED WHITEFISH.—After the fish has been cleaned, cut in pieces and put in a weak brine for an hour or more. When wanted take from salt water, and dry in towel, dip the pieces in beaten egg and then in corn meal and drop in hot lard as you would doughnuts. The lard may be kept to use again as in frying cakes.

CODFISH A LA MODE.—Teacup codfish picked up fine, two cups of mashed potatoes, one pint of cream or milk, two eggs well beaten, half cup of butter, salt and pepper; mix well, bake in baking dish from twenty to twenty-five minutes.

BAKED WHITEFISH.—Take fish, rub inside and outside with salt and pepper, fill with stuffing made like that for poultry, sew up and put in hot pan with part drippings and part butter; dredge with flour and lay over fish a few thin slices of bacon. In baking, allow twenty-five minutes to a pound of fish; baste occasionally.

CODFISH BALLS.—Take two parts of mashed .potatoes to one of picked codfish which has been previously freshened, and one beaten egg; mix well together and make in cakes and fry in butter, or in balls the size of a walnut, and drop in hot lard and fry a light brown. They are much nicer by dipping in egg and then in cracker crumbs before frying.

Fish Turbot.—Steam fresh whitefish until you can take the bones out; pick to pieces, then make a dressing of a pint of milk thickened with quarter pound of flour; when cool add two well beaten eggs and one quarter pound of butter, put in baking dish, alternate layers of fish and sauce until filled, cover top with bread or cracker crumbs and bake half an hour.

Escalloped Fish.—Pick any cold fresh fish, or salt codfish, left from the dinner, into fine bits, carefully removing all the bones. Take a pint of milk in a suitable dish, and place it in a saucepan of boiling water; put into it a few slices of onion, cut very fine, a sprig of parsley minced fine, add a piece of butter as large as an egg, a pinch of salt, a sprinkle of white pepper; then stir in two tablespoonfuls of cornstarch, or flour rubbed in a little cold milk. Let all boil up and remove from the fire. Take a dish you wish to serve it in, butter the sides and bottom. Put first a layer of the minced fish, then a layer of the cream, then sprinkle over that some cracker or bread crumbs, then a layer of fish again, and so on, until the dish is full. Spread cracker or bread crumbs last on top, to prevent the milk from scorching. Nice breakfast or side dish at dinner.

Salmon Turbot.—One can salmon, three eggs beaten light, four tablespoons melted butter, half cup fine bread crumbs; season with salt, pepper and parsley. Beat fish and butter together until smooth. Beat bread crumbs and eggs together, then put all together. Put in buttered mould and steam one hour. Sauce for turbot: One cup milk heated to boiling, thickened with one tablespoon cornstarch, the juice from the salmon, one large spoonful of butter, one teaspoon catsup, a little parsley and pepper, and one egg beaten and put in last. Then very carefully let all just come to boiling. Serve on hot platter and pour sauce over the turbot just before sending to the table.—*Mrs. Edward Cahill.*

TURBOT.—Steam a whitefish until tender, remove from the bones while hot, and season with pepper and salt. Turbot dressing: One quart of milk, three slices of onions, and a little parsley. When it comes to a boil, take out the onion and parsley and put in a quarter pound of butter, pepper and salt, half a cup of flour; stir until smooth. Let it cool for ten or fifteen minutes. When cool stir in two well beaten eggs. Put in a layer of dressing with bread crumbs grated over the top. Bake twenty minutes in a hot oven.—*Mrs. F. B. Lee.*

SALMON TURBOT.—One cup of milk, two teaspoons of flour and a little butter cooked together. Two eggs beaten in after this is taken from the stove. Mix with a can of salmon and bake.—*Mrs. Earle.*

CODFISH BALLS, No. 1.—Shred cold boiled codfish very fine, add to it an equal or even more of mashed potatoes, moisten with one beaten egg or two or three tablespoonfuls of sweet milk. Season with pepper and a little butter. Make small flat cakes, flour and fry brown in drippings or lard.—*Mrs. Geo. Ritter.*

CODFISH BALLS, No. 2.—Pick up as fine as possible a teacup of nice white codfish. Freshen all night, or, if wanted for any other meal than breakfast, from the morning, scald it once and drain off the water; chop and work until entirely fine. Put it in a basin with water, a bit of butter the size of an egg, and two eggs; beat it thoroughly and heat it until it thickens, without boiling. It should, when all is mixed, be about a quart. Have some potatoes ready prepared and nicely mashed, work the fish and potatoes thoroughly together as above, make it in flat cakes, and brown on both sides. This is a very nice dish, as all who have tried will allow.

SALMON.—Take one cup of salmon, pour off the oil, put on a warm platter, and take out the bones. Set in a hot oven for a few minutes. Take out and cover with drawn butter. Serve while hot.—*Mrs. H. R. Pratt.*

LOBSTER RISOLES.—Extract the meat of a boiled lobster, mince it fine as possible, mix with it the coral pounded smooth, and the yolks of two hard-boiled eggs. Season high with cayenne pepper, powdered mace and salt. Mix a batter of beaten eggs, milk and flour, allowing to each egg two tablespoons of milk and one teaspoon of flour. Beat the batter well, then mix in the lobster gradually, till stiff enough to make into oval balls the size of a large plum. Fry in butter. Serve hot or cold.—*Mrs. F. B. Lee.*

HOT SALMON.—Two cans of salmon, three well beaten eggs. Season with butter, salt and pepper, press in a bowl and steam one-half hour. Turn on a platter and pour over the following sauce: One pint of milk, boiled; stir in one tablespoon of flour, one tablespoon of butter, and just before serving add one beaten egg.—*Mrs. J. L. Parker, Dowagiac.*

SALMON LOAF.—One small can salmon, four eggs beaten separately, four tablespoonfuls butter melted, but not hot, one-half cup fine bread crumbs. Season with pepper, salt and minced parsley. Chop fish fine, then rub butter in until smooth. Beat crumbs into eggs and season before working together. Put into buttered mold and steam one hour. Dressing: One cup of milk, heated to a boil, thicken with one tablespoonful cornstarch and one of butter rubbed together, then put in the liquor of the salmon, one egg and a little pepper. Put the egg in last and very carefully add a little chopped parsley. —*Mrs. L. C. Storrs.*

OYSTERS.

Plain Oyster Soup.—Drain the liquor from one quart of oysters and to it add one quart of boiling water, let boil and skim thoroughly, season with butter and pepper to taste, add oysters, let come to boiling heat; season with salt and serve.

Oyster Soup with Milk.—Pour one-half pint cold water over one quart of oysters, drain through a colander into a soup kettle, add one quart of milk, let come to a boil and skim; season with pepper, add oysters, allowing them to come to a boil, add salt, pour upon bits of butter in tureen and serve.—*Mrs. N. B. Jones.*

Individual Baked Oysters.—Drain the liquor from a quart of oysters into a porcelain kettle and when it boils put in the oysters. Have a tablespoonful of flour rubbed well into two tablespoonfuls of butter. When the oysters swell stir in the butter and flour. Cook until the oysters are white and plump; then add a half cup cream, pepper and salt. Put into oyster shells, sprinkle with cracker crumbs and little butter. Bake a nice brown and serve in the shells. —*Mrs. L. Hudson.*

Oyster Pie.—Make a crust the same as for chicken pie, and after lining a dish with it, put in a layer of oysters. Butter, pepper and salt these, then put in another layer of oysters and do likewise. Thicken a little of the strained oyster liquor with flour and pour over the top. Cover with crust and bake until a nice brown.—*Kittie Walker.*

Broiled Oysters.—Drain select oysters in a colander; dip them, one by one, in melted butter, to prevent their sticking to the gridiron; have the iron hot before placing them upon it; broil over a clear fire. When nicely brown on both sides season with salt, pepper and butter, and lay them on hot, buttered toast.—*Mrs. Earle.*

OYSTER PATTIES.—Make a rich puff paste and line little pans and bake a light brown. Take one pint of milk, two tablespoons of flour, one tablespoon of butter, a little salt, and stir in the milk while boiling. Throw in more than half a can of oysters and let them scald, then put in an oyster or two with some of the liquor into each pattie. Serve while hot. Same patties may be filled with jelly.—*Mrs. F. B. Lee.*

OYSTER TOAST.—One cup cream, one can oysters, one tablespoon flour rubbed in butter and put in the boiling cream. Take the oysters from the juice and put them in the boiling mixture. When they just boil pour over buttered toast.—*Kate T. Cooley.*

OYSTER ROLLS.—One and one-half pints oysters chopped; one and one-half pounds cooked veal chopped; two tablespoonfuls butter; nine tablespoonfuls cracker crumbs; yolks of three eggs; salt and pepper. Make into balls, then roll in cracker crumbs and fry in hot lard. (Rolls more delicate if all oysters instead of part veal.)—*Mrs. J. N. Alexander.*

ESCALLOPED OYSTERS.—Butter a pudding dish and sprinkle a layer of cracker or bread crumbs in the bottom of the dish; then a layer of oysters with bits of butter, pepper and salt; then a layer of crumbs, and so on until the dish is full, with crumbs and bits of butter on top. Then add to the oyster liquor its measure of milk or cream, with the addition of a beaten egg. Put in oven and bake half an hour.—*Mrs. E. A. Gilkey.*

LITTLE PIGS IN BLANKETS.—Eighteen large oysters, bacon and toast Wrap each oyster in a slice of thin bacon, and fasten with wooden toothpicks. Put the little pigs in a pan; turn constantly until they are brown. Serve on toast.—*Mrs. Chester Brown, Lake Charles, La.*

Oyster Potpie.—Scald a quart can of oysters in their own liquor; when it boils, skim out the oysters and set aside in a warm place. To the liquor add a pint of hot water; season well with salt and pepper, a generous piece of butter, thicken with flour and cold milk. Have ready nice light biscuit dough, rolled twice as thick as pie crust; cut into inch squares, drop them into the boiling stew, cover closely and cook forty minutes. When taken up, stir the oysters into the juice and serve all together in one dish. A nice side entree.

Receipt for Hash.—Hash is made out ov kast off vittles, homogenius abnormal, and at times uneak in its natur. Hash has dun more to push the human family than any other kind of mixt phood. It will be impossible to lay down enny specifik rule to kreate this abstruse, and at the same time gentle phood. Ennything that will chop fluently will produce hash. No one has taken out a patent yet for the production of this permiskious viand. Hash requires but little cooking, but may be compared to a foundered horse—goes best when well warmed up. For the kreashun of hash, tallent is ov more importance than genius. Finally, hash may be likened to the human family—from sum standpoints it is fair, from others it is bad, and from all suspicious.—*Josh Billings.*

MEAT, POULTRY AND GAME.

"You may make houses enchantingly beautiful, have them clean, airy and convenient, but if the stomach is fed with sour bread and burnt meats, it will raise such rebellion, that the eyes will see no beauty anywhere."

HINTS FOR COOKING MEATS.

If you would preserve all the nutriment in fresh meat do not place in cold water; place in boiling water and cook gently. Hard boiling toughens it.

When broiling steak give it your undivided attention. Turn often and do not season while cooking.

Singe poultry with alcohol.

A scant teaspoon of sugar added to meat gravy gives a delicious flavor.

In roasting meat place dry in the pan, do not season or put water in the dripper for thirty minutes after placing in a very hot oven, It is a prevalent idea that meat will burn in roasting, if not basted or wet with drippings, the fact is meat will bear all the heat necessary to roast it in the most perfect manner, and not burn. Resting dry upon the bottom of the pan, upper and under sides brown evenly at the same time; and not only is the process of roasting shortened. but nearly all the trouble of changing the positions of the meat in the oven is avoided.

Baked Ham.—Soak a ten-pound ham over night in plenty of cold water. In the morning scrape clean and wipe dry. To five pounds of flour add enough cold water to make a stiff dough. Roll this out about one inch thick and cover the ham with it. Place it in a baking pan with the fat side up, and bake steadily for five hours. Should the crust slip off, leaving parts of the ham exposed, mend with flour and water When the ham is cooked, break off the crust, skin the ham, sprinkle with brown sugar, and brown in a quick oven.

How to Use Cold Steak.—Take pieces of cold steak or meat, chop fine; soak three or more slices of bread in some sweet milk, mash fine; one egg beaten. Mix all together, season to taste and drop with a spoon into hot butter, and fry brown.

Beefsteak.—Have a clear bed of glowing coals. The steak should be about three-quarters of an inch in thickness, and should be pounded only in extreme cases, *i. e.*, when it is cut too thick and is "stringy." Lay it on a buttered gridiron, turning it often as it begins to drip, attempting nothing else while cooking it. Have everything else ready for the table; the potatoes and vegetables dished and in the warming closet. Do not season it until it is done, which will be in about ten to twelve minutes. Remove it to a warm platter, pepper and salt it on both sides and spread a liberal lump of butter over it. Serve at once while hot. No definite rule can be given as to the *time* of cooking steak, individual tastes differ so widely in regard to it. The best pieces for broiling are the porter-house and sirloin.

Pot-Roast of Beef.—Have your kettle hot, into it put your beef, turning until seared over the outside; then pour in a pint of boiling water and boil rapidly for ten minutes, salt, cover closely and set back where it will simmer gently for four hours. Before serving, draw forward, remove the cover to let the water evaporate, and brown slightly.—*Mrs. Chas. M. Turner.*

Beefsteak Rolls.—Prepare a good dressing, such as you like for turkey or duck; take a round steak, pound it, but not very hard, spread the dressing over it, sprinkle in a little salt, pepper, and a few bits of butter, lap over the ends, roll the steak up tightly and tie closely; spread two great spoonfuls of butter over the steak after rolling it up, then wash with a well-beaten egg, put water in the bake-pan, lay in the steak so as not to touch the water, and bake as you would a duck, basting often. A half hour in a brisk oven will bake. Make a brown gravy, and send to the table hot.

English Pickle for Tongue.—For two tongues, make a brine of two ounces of salt-petre, one-half pound of brown sugar, one pint of barrel salt, one cupful of molasses, water enough to cover them. Let them stand in a crock, well kept under the brine for ten days. This brine can be used as long as it will keep sweet.—*Saginaw Cook Book.*

Beef Stew.—Three pounds beef and a calf's foot. (Have your butcher chop the foot in small pieces.) Take one tablespoon of butter, two of flour, and place in a dripper or shallow pan on top of the stove, stirring it until a light brown; to this add one pint of boiling water. Then wash the beef and put in the pan, placing the calf's foot around it. Add one onion, with two cloves, one carrot, one teaspoon of salt and one-half teaspoon of pepper. Cover the pan so that no steam escapes and let it simmer for five hours. The expense of this dish is twenty-five cents, and it is delicious.—*Mrs. C. C. Wood.*

Beefsteak Toast.—Chop cold steak very fine, cook in a little water, put in cream or milk, thicken, season with butter, salt and pepper, and pour it over slices of toast. Prepare boiled ham in the same way, adding the yolk of an egg.—*Mrs. C. J. Davis.*

Veal Collops.—Cut veal from the leg or other lean part into pieces the size of an oyster. Season with pepper, salt and a little mace; rub some over each piece; dip in egg, then in cracker crumbs, and fry. They both look and taste like oysters.

VEAL PATTIES.—Cut portions of the neck or breast of veal into small pieces, and with a little salt pork cut fine, stew gently for ten or fifteen minutes, season with pepper and salt and a small piece of celery chopped coarsely, also of the yellow top, picked (not chopped) up; stir in a paste made of a tablespoonful of flour, the yolk of one egg, and milk to form a thin batter; let all come to a boil and it is ready for the patties. Make the patties of a light, flaky crust, as for tarts, cut round, the size of a small sauce plate, the center of each, for about three inches, cut half way through, to be raised and serve as a cover. Put a spoonful of the stew in each crust, lay on the top, and serve. Stewed oysters or lamb may be used in place of veal.

FOR COOKING VEAL CUTLETS.—Beat the veal until it is almost broken to shreds. Have eggs (as many as necessary) beaten; have some crackers rolled and seasoned with salt and pepper; dip the veal first into the egg, then into the crackers. Have your lard very hot and drop your cutlet into it. The hot lard draws the meat together again, and when done it will be as tender as chicken.—*Mrs. Pres. Harrison in Wimodausis Cook Book.*

VEAL LOAF.—Two pounds veal chopped fine, one cup rolled crackers, butter size of an egg, two eggs, one tablespoon salt, one teaspoon pepper, one cup milk. Bake two hours.—*Mrs. W. E. Trager.*

STEAMED LEG OF MUTTON.—Wash and put the leg in a steamer and cook it until tender, then place in a roasting pan, salt and dredge well with flour and set in a hot oven until nicely browned. Serve with currant jelly.

FRIED MUTTON CHOPS.—Prepare by trimming off all extra fat and skin, season with salt and pepper; dip each chop in beaten egg, then in rolled cracker or bread crumbs; dip again in the egg and crumbs, and so on until they are well coated with the crumbs. Have ready a deep spider containing a pound or more of lard, hot enough to fry crullers. Drop into this hot lard the chops, frying only a few at one time, as too many cool the fat. Fry them brown, and serve up hot and dry on a warm platter.

MUTTON CUTLETS (BAKED).—Prepare same as for frying, lay them in a dripping pan with a very little water in the bottom. Bake quickly, and baste often with butter and water. Make a little brown gravy and turn over them when they are served.

BREADED SPRING CHICKEN.—Cut spring chicken into pieces, dip first into beaten egg, then into grated bread crumbs; season with minced parsley, pepper and salt; place in a pan, lay bits of butter over, add a little water, set in the oven and bake slowly, basting often.

INDIVIDUAL CHICKEN PIES.—Put one pint milk in porcelain kettle; when boiling add one tablespoonful of flour which has been well rubbed into two tablespoonfuls of butter, then add cold chicken cut into small pieces. Season with salt, pepper and a little curry. Line your tins with good puff paste, rather thinner than paste for top, bake a nice brown and serve hot.—*Mrs. L. S. Hudson.*

TWICE LAID.—Cut up or chop cold chicken in small pieces, put these in a buttered baking-dish, sprinkle with flour and season well. Moisten with cream or milk, but if milk is used add butter. Any remnant of gravy or stock is an improvement. The chicken should be quite moist. Take cold boiled rice, thin it with milk so that it can be spread easily over the meat, about an inch in thickness. Put bits of butter over the top and bake for half an hour.—*Mrs. C. J. Davis.*

CREAMED CHICKEN.—One chicken, if 4½ lbs., or two of 6 lbs., four sweetbreads, and one can of mushrooms. Boil chicken and sweetbreads, and when cold cut up as for salad. In a saucepan put four coffee cups, or one quart of cream; in another put four large tablespoons butter and five even ones of flour; stir until melted. Then pour in the hot cream, stirring until it thickens; flavor with a small half of grated onion and a very little grated nutmeg; season highly with black and red pepper. Put chicken and ingredients together with sweetbreads and mushrooms (which if large should be cut in four pieces) in a baking dish, cover with bread crumbs and pieces of butter, and bake 20 minutes. Serves sixteen persons.—*Miss Flora Buck.*

Chicken Patties.—Mince up fine cold chicken, either roasted or boiled. Season it with pepper and salt and a little minced parsley and onion. Moisten it with chicken gravy or cream sauce; fill scalloped shells that are lined with pastry with the mixture, and sprinkle bread crumbs over the tops. Put two or three tiny pieces of butter over each, and bake brown in a hot oven.

Baked Calf's Heart.—Wash off the blood, stuff with a stuffing as for turkey. Tie a buttered paper over the mouth of the heart to keep the stuffing in place. Put it in a small baking pan with a little hot water, pepper and salt. Bake nearly two hours, basting it very frequently. When done, thicken the gravy with flour and serve. It is really nice to be sliced and eaten cold.—*Mrs. F. B. Lee.*

Stuffed Liver.—Soak a calf's liver in salted water an hour or more, changing once. Make a stuffing of bread crumbs and a little chopped salt pork, seasoned highly with pepper, salt and summer savory. Make incisions in the liver and fill them with the stuffing, then roll and tie it. Blanket with slices of salt pork, and either boil or bake it. To be eaten cold for lunch or tea.—*Mrs. F. B. Lee.*

Veal Loaf.—Three and one-half pounds of lean veal (not cooked) and one-half pound of salt pork chopped very fine; mix with it six soda crackers rolled fine, three well-beaten eggs, one tablespoon salt, one-half teaspoon of pepper, four tablespoons of cream, milk or water; butter the size of an egg. Mix thoroughly, make into a loaf; put in a dripping pan with enough hot water to baste. Bake from two to three hours. It can also be made with beef.—*Mrs. C. F. Swift.*

BEEF OR VEAL LOAF.—Three pounds meat, chopped fine, two eggs, one and one-half cups crackers (rolled), a heaping tablespoon butter, pepper, salt, and half a cup water. Bake two and one-half hours.—*Mrs. Roxie Donovan.*

VEAL LOAF.—Four pounds of raw chopped veal and one pound of salt pork, one cup of rolled crackers, one egg well beaten, pepper and salt and sage to suit taste.—*Mrs. J. M. Earle.*

Meat loaves are much improved by being occasionally dripped with slightly salted water.

SCALLOPED MEAT.—Chop meat very fine, mash with masher until smooth. To one cup of meat add three-fourths pint of boiling milk, four tablespoons of butter, two tablespoons cornstarch, one-half teaspoon salt, one-half saltspoon of black pepper. Melt butter, lifting often from stove; put cornstarch into melted butter. As soon as it begins to boil, add boiling milk, a little at a time, until butter and cornstarch are perfectly smooth. Then mix meat into this and let cool. Put it into shells, sprinkle over them rolled cracker crumbs seasoned with melted butter—use plenty of crumbs. Set shells into a dripper with a little boiling water in bottom and bake.—*Mrs. J. E. Nichols.*

MOCK DUCK.—Take a round of beefsteak, salt and pepper it; prepare a dressing as for turkey, lay your dressing on the meat, sew up, and roast one-half hour. Put water in the pan with plenty of butter and a sliced onion, baste frequently. Thicken the gravy with a little flour rubbed smooth.—*Mrs. F. B. Lee.*

FRIZZLED DRIED BEEF.—Cut your beef very thin, then pull it into small pieces, taking out all the strings of sinew, fat, and bits of outside; put it in the frying pan, and cover with cold water; let it simmer on the back part of the stove till perfectly tender; then pour off the water, and cover the beef with cream; add pepper, celery-salt, and salt if needed. Mix one tablespoonful of melted butter, with one heaped tablespoon of flour, and stir into the hot cream; cover and keep very hot till served.

TENDERLOIN ON TOAST.—Cut pork tenderloins in very thin slices; stew them in a little water till they are done; then put a little butter in a saucepan, and fry them till light brown. Serve on buttered toast and raw tomatoes sliced thin.

HAM TOAST.—Chop lean cooked ham into small pieces; put in a pan with a little pepper, a lump of butter and two eggs well beaten. When warm through spread on buttered toast.—*Mrs. J. E. Nichols.*

DUMPLINGS FOR POTPIE.—Take a small teacup of flour, a pinch of salt, one and one-half teaspoons of baking powder, butter size of a walnut, sprinkle in a little pepper, add sweet milk enough to form a stiff dough; flour the board, roll thinner than biscuit; cut in small squares; drop in soup or broth. Boil ten minutes.

VEAL OMELET.—Chop fine two pounds of veal, roll a half dozen crackers and mix with the veal; add two eggs, a little chopped parsley, and salt and pepper. Make into a roll and bake. Baste with butter and milk while baking.

FRIED SWEETBREADS.—Thoroughly clean the sweetbreads, remove the gristle, and lay in salt and water two hours. Parboil them, throw them into cold water to harden them. Cut into slices not too thin, and fry in hot lard. If prepared, a batter can be made with beaten eggs and flour in which the sweetbreads can be dipped before frying. —*Mrs. F. B. Lee.*

Smothered Beefsteak.—Take round steak, cut about one inch thick. Lay it in a dripping pan and sprinkle thick with cracker crumbs, put bits of butter on the top, season to suit the taste, moisten with hot water, set in a hot oven and bake one hour.

Escalloped Chicken.—One chicken boiled and cut as for salad. Make a dressing of one cup of cream, one egg, one tablespoon cornstarch, piece of butter size of an egg. Boil cream and butter together, add cornstarch wet with a little cold milk, then add egg, chicken, salt and pepper. Butter the dish, sprinkle the bottom with bread crumbs and pieces of butter. Bake twenty-eight minutes or until brown. Nice for a dinner course.—*Mrs. G. L. Freeman.*

Broiled Venison Steak.—Venison steak should be broiled over a clear fire, turning often. It requires more cooking than beef. When sufficiently done, season with salt and pepper, pour over two tablespoonfuls of currant jelly, melted with a piece of butter. Serve hot on hot plates.

Roast Quail.—Rinse well and steam over boiling water until tender, then dredge with flour and smother in butter; season with salt and pepper and roast inside the stove; thicken the gravy; serve with green grape jelly and garnish with parsley.

Roast Partridge.—Clean and wash the birds, draw into position and tie firmly with twine. Salt and rub the breast and legs with soft butter, dredge thickly with flour, put into a quick oven and bake forty minutes. If liked rare, twenty-five minutes will suffice. When done place on a hot dish on which has been placed bread crumbs. Garnish with parsley and serve with a bread sauce.

BREAD SAUCE FOR GAME.—Two cups of milk, one of dried crumbs, a quarter of an onion, two tablespoons butter, and salt and pepper. Dry the bread in a warm oven, and roll into rather coarse crumbs. Sift, and put the fine crumbs which come through and which make about a third of a cupful on to boil with the milk and onions. Boil ten or fifteen minutes and add a tablespoon of butter and seasoning. Skim out the onions. Fry the coarse crumbs a light brown in the remaining butter, which must be very hot before they are put in. Stir over a hot fire two minutes, being watchful not to burn. Cover the breasts of the roasted birds with these, and serve the sauce poured round the birds or in a gravy dish.—*Mrs. Chas. M. Turner.*

SADDLE OF VENISON.—Venison should be soaked in weak vinegar over night, highly seasoned with salt and red pepper. Before cooking, lard very thoroughly with salt pork. I will explain for the benefit of young housekeepers that this is done by cutting slits in the meat in which you insert the salt pork. Larding needles are sold for this purpose, but are not necessary. After taking out of the vinegar rub with salt and a little red pepper. Venison should be roasted and well done. Currant jelly can be added to the gravy.—*Mrs. Jas. M. Turner.*

PARTRIDGE AND QUAIL.—Skin the birds and split down the back. Unless the birds have hung for some time they should be kept in a cool place several days before cooking. Cover the breasts with slices of salt pork and roast in the oven from twenty to thirty minutes. Quail should always be served on crisp toast. Both partridge and quail can have a cream sauce for gravy if desired. Currant jelly should be served with all roasted game.—*Mrs. Jas. M. Turner.*

WILD DUCKS.—Pluck the feathers without scalding. These birds should never be skinned as there is a heavy layer of fat under the skin which pulls off with it, and when denuded of this fat the meat of a wild duck is dry and unpalatable. Singe very carefully with alcohol flame or burning paper. Then take out the entrails and wash in cold water. After standing for a time to drain, wipe dry inside and out, and keep several days in a cool place if the birds are freshly killed—in very cold weather a week or ten days. Ducks are best, roasted, and stuffed with a dressing made of dry bread crumbs, with a large quantity of finely-chopped onion added. It should be further seasoned with salt, black pepper and melted butter. It must be remembered that connoisseurs like game cooked very rare. In view of this, when birds are prepared for such people, twenty minutes in the oven will be sufficient. I find, however, that most people like game well done, and a good sized duck should be roasted one hour. Experience assures me that all game, poultry and meats are best roasted in a covered baker. Before putting the ducks in the oven rub inside and out with a little red pepper and plenty of salt. A little water in the pan as you begin roasting is desirable. The giblets can be boiled, chopped very fine, and added to the gravy, which should be thickened with flour stirred smooth in water. Currant jelly, if desired, can be added to the gravy immediately before serving.—*Mrs. Jas. M. Turner.*

VENISON.—Take a haunch of venison, put in a large kettle, cover with water, and boil until tender; drain off the water, put one-half pound of butter with salt and pepper into the kettle, set over a moderate fire and let brown, first on one side and then on the other. Venison cooked in this way retains its natural flavor, and will be found delicious.—*Old Kentucky Huntsman's Receipt.*

'A commonplace life," we say and we sigh,
  But why should we sigh as we say?
The commonplace sun in the commonplace sky
  Makes up the commonplace day.
The moon and the stars are commonplace things,
  And the flower that blooms and the bird that sings.
But dark were the world, and sad our lot,
  If the flowers should fail and the sun shine not—
And God, who studies each separate soul,
  Out of commonplace lives makes his beautiful whole."
—*Susan Coolidge.*

All Good Housekeepers Know

How much depends on the Oven.

With a **GAS RANGE**——
you have the heat completely under control.

Gas for Fuel . . .
is SAFE, CLEAN and ECONOMICAL.

Gas Stoves . . .
are REASONABLE IN PRICE.

Inquire of one of the many ladies using them,
or see samples at the office.

——LANSING GAS LIGHT CO.

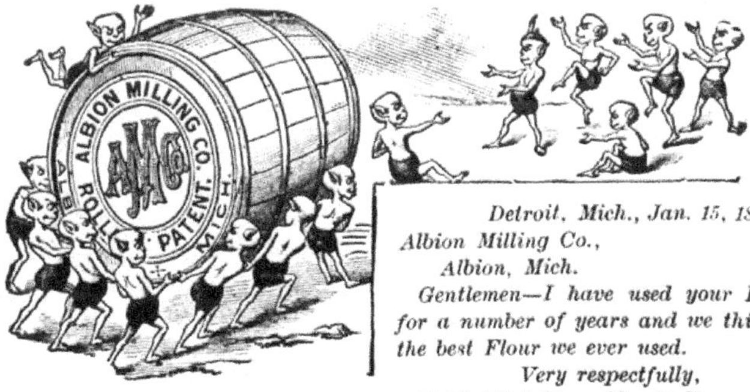

Detroit, Mich., Jan. 15, 1895.
Albion Milling Co.,
Albion, Mich.
Gentlemen—I have used your Flour for a number of years and we think it the best Flour we ever used.
Very respectfully,
26 W. High St. Mrs. S. Brownell,

CROQUETTES.

Oyster Croquettes.—Twenty-five oysters, or one can of oysters and their liquor, one gill of cream, one tablespoonful of butter, two tablespoonfuls of flour, one tablespoonful of chopped parsley, yolks of two eggs, one-fourth of nutmeg grated, salt and cayenne pepper to taste. Put the oysters to boil in their own liquor, boil and stir constantly for five minutes; then take from fire, drain, and chop very fine. Now put into a saucepan one gill of this liquor and cream. Rub together the butter and the flour, add this and the oysters to the boiling liquor and cream and stir until it boils and thickens. Now add the yolks of the eggs, stir over fire one minute, take off and add parsley, salt, cayenne and nutmeg. Mix well and turn out to cool. When cold form into croquettes, roll first in beaten egg, then in bread crumbs and fry in boiling oil or fat.

Sweet Potato Croquettes.—Boil six large potatoes until tender. Then remove the skins and mash the potatoes through a colander. Add one tablespoonful of butter, one teaspoonful of salt, one of sugar and a dash of pepper. Mix all thoroughly and form into croquettes. Dip first in egg, then in bread crumbs, and fry in smoking hot lard.

Rice Croquettes.—Boil one-half cup of milk and stir into it one cup of cold boiled rice, one tablespoonful of butter, and one-half teaspoonful of salt. When it boils add one egg, well beaten, and cook two minutes longer. When cold make into rolls or balls, dip in egg and cracker crumbs and fry.

Salmon Croquettes.—One can salmon chopped fine, three fine rolled crackers of large size, a pinch of pepper and salt, and one egg. Roll in crackers, fry in boiling lard, and serve with mayonnaise made as follows: Yolks of three eggs, stir well with one scant tablespoon of granulated sugar, pinch of salt, one tablespoonful of mustard dissolved in vinegar, one-half tablespoonful butter. Stir all well and cook in double steamer. Add one-half cup vinegar and one-half cup sweet cream.

LOBSTER CROQUETTES.—Chop the meat of a well-boiled lobster, add pepper and salt. Mix this with one-fourth as much bread crumbs as you have meat; with two tablespoonfuls of melted butter and yolks of two eggs, form into balls. Roll these in beaten egg, then in cracker crumbs and fry in hot deep lard.—*Mrs. L. H.*

FISH CROQUETTES.—One tablespoon butter, one heaping tablespoon flour, one cup milk (or water), one cup cold flaked fish, one egg. Season with salt and pepper and a dash of onion. Rub the flour and butter together, add to it over the fire the milk or water, and when thick add fish. Let it boil up once, then take from fire; break in an egg and stir thoroughly. Season with salt and pepper; set away to cool. Then roll into cork shaped croquettes, roll in fine cracker crumbs, then in beaten egg, and again in cracker crumbs and fry in boiling lard. Serve on a napkin.—*Mrs. Edward Cahill.*

CHICKEN CROQUETTES.—Take any kind of fresh meat or fowl, chop very fine, add an equal quantity of smoothly mashed potatoes, mix and season with butter, salt, black pepper, a little prepared mustard, and a little cayenne pepper; make into cakes, dip in eggs and bread crumbs and fry a light brown. A nice relish for tea.

VEAL CROQUETTES.—Mince a coffee cup of cold veal in a chopping bowl, add a little cold ham and two or three slices of onion, a pinch of mace, powdered parsley and pepper, some salt. Let a pint of milk or cream come to the boiling point, then add a tablespoonful of cold butter, then the above mixture. Beat up two eggs and mix with a teaspoonful of cornstarch or flour, and add to the rest. Cook it all about ten minutes, stirring with care. Remove from the fire, and spread it on a platter, roll it into balls; when cooled flatten each; dip in egg and bread crumbs, and fry in a wire basket, dipped in hot lard.

Chicken Croquettes, No. 1.—One-half pound chicken chopped fine seasoned with one-fourth teaspoon of salt, one-half teaspoon cayenne pepper, one teaspoon lemon juice, one-fourth teaspoon white pepper. Mix with a white cream sauce, roll in fine bread crumbs, dip in egg, then in crumbs again, and fry. Sauce is made by heating one and one-half tablespoons of butter until bubbling; stir in three heaping tablespoons of flour dry and when well mixed add a scant pint of milk, celery, salt and pepper, and boil until as thick as butter.

Chicken Croquettes, No. 2.—One solid pint of finely chopped cooked chicken or other meat. One tablespoon of salt, one-half teaspoon of pepper, one cupful of cream or chicken stock, one tablespoon of flour, four eggs, one tablespoon of onion juice, one tablespoon of butter. Put the cream or stock on to boil, mix flour and butter together and stir into cream, then add rest and boil two minutes, then add two of the eggs well beaten. When cool, shape and roll in cracker crumbs, and fry in hot lard.

Potato Croquettes.—Two cups hot mashed potatoes; one tablespoon butter; salt to taste; two yolks of eggs beaten light; one teaspoon chopped parsley; dust of cayenne pepper; two tablespoons sweet cream; one teaspoon onion juice. Stir this mixture over the fire until it will not stick to the pan (about five minutes.) For wetting: whites of one egg, one tablespoon of hot water; stir just enough to mix; must not froth; dip in this then roll in cracker crumbs; fry in very hot lard; will cook in one minute. This will make one dozen.—*Mrs. C. J. Davis.*

SALADS.

Success in cooking comes from skill, not chance. In making salads, have everything as cold as possible, and all materials of the freshest. Salads should be stirred lightly with a fork, never packed. "Salads are wholesome food as well as dainty relishes; and their value among all classes as hygienic and esthetic agents can scarcely be overestimated. They are so inexpensive, easily made, and require so little thought or labor; they utilize so many odds and ends of food frequently permitted to go to waste, that their general introduction would be a national blessing."

Salad Dressing Without Oil.—One slightly heaping tablespoonful of mustard mixed with a little hot water, one-half cupful vinegar, three eggs well beaten; set in the top of a teakettle, and cook to consistency of custard. Strain through wire sieve, and allow it to become perfectly cold before using. Before pouring over salad, thin with cream. This is good for chicken, or any salad.—*Mrs. C. J. Davis.*

Salad Dressing.—Well-beaten yolks of five eggs, five tablespoons of very sour vinegar, two even teaspoons of mustard, two even teaspoons salt, one teaspoon sugar, one sprinkling red pepper. Cook in a farina boiler stirring all the while until moderately thick. Remove from fire and add one-half cup of butter in a fine thread-like stream, beating the mixture rapidly all the while; it should be very smooth. Be careful and not cook too much or it will be too thick. If you want it extra fine strain the mixture before cooking to get out all the little lumps. Just before making salad add a cup of sweet cream to every cup of dressing.—*Miss Alice Daily.*

SALAD DRESSING THAT WILL KEEP.—One cup of vinegar, small half cup of sugar, four eggs, one teaspoon of flour, one teaspoon of mustard. Let vinegar and sugar come to a boil, add beaten eggs slowly, then flour wet with a little water, then mustard and a small piece of butter. When wanted for use add sweet cream to thin.—*Mrs. Fred. S. Lawrence.*

SALAD DRESSING.—Yolks of four eggs creamed with two heaping tablespoons of sugar and one even teaspoon of mustard and a pinch of salt; add a lump of butter size of a walnut, then put in six tablespoons of vinegar and six tablespoons of milk. Cook over hot water. —*Mrs. J. P. Edmonds.*

SALAD CREAM DRESSING.—One and one-half tablespoons of dry American mustard, one teaspoon of salt, a little pepper, scald with hot water enough to mix. Use melted butter or olive oil; drop it in slowly, all it will take up; put in three eggs and beat all together. Add one-half cup of vinegar and two-thirds of a cup of milk; put it on the stove, bringing to a boil, stirring constantly. Very nice and will keep a long time.—*Mrs. W. S. Griswold.*

SALAD DRESSING.—Yolks of four eggs, one-half cup of butter, one cup of vinegar. Heat butter and vinegar and pour boiling hot on eggs well beaten.—*Mrs. John Rork.*

SALAD DRESSING.—One cup of vinegar, two tablespoons of flour, one tablespoon of butter, one egg, one and one-half teaspoons of salt, one-half teaspoon of black pepper, three teaspoons of mustard, a pinch of cayenne. Beat all together, and stir while cooking. When cooled add one cup of cream or rich milk and beat thoroughly —*Mrs. Geo. Ritter.*

POTATO SALAD.—Take four large cold boiled potatoes, cut them in slices and stew with cream or milk and butter, seasoning them as for eating. Make a salad dressing of the yolks of four eggs beaten, a teaspoonful of powdered white sugar, a saltspoon of cayenne, two teaspoonfuls of made mustard, two tablespoonfuls of vinegar and four tablespoonfuls of salad oil.—*Mrs. F. B. Lee.*

CABBAGE SALAD. — Two eggs, one-half cup vinegar, four tablespoonfuls sugar, butter the size of a hickory nut, small teaspoon flour, little salt. Beat all together and boil, then set to cool; then add one cup sour cream and beat until light, then pour over the cabbage.—*Mrs. R. B. Kellogg.*

TOMATO SALAD.—One quart canned tomatoes, one-quarter box gelatine; pass the tomatoes through a sieve and season; stiffen with the gelatine, which has been previously melted, pour into small, round molds. Serve on lettuce leaves with salad dressing.—*Miss Cornelia A. Sibbald, Saginaw.*

NUT SALAD.—Two cups of cut celery, one cup of English walnuts chopped fine. Pour over this a mayonnaise dressing to which sour cream has been added. Serve on lettuce.—*Mrs. Chas. Shubel.*

TOMATO AND CUCUMBER SALAD.—Two raw tomatoes, one cucumber, one-half box of gelatine. Soak gelatine, chop vegetables and season with salt, pepper, vinegar and a dash of onion; mix with gelatine. When the jelly hardens, turn out on fresh lettuce leaves and pour over a mayonnaise. The mould may be lined with thin slices of cucumber if desired.—*Mrs. C. J. Davis.*

POTATO SALAD.—Sliced potatoes, onions and cucumbers, salt and pepper. Pour over the following dressing: One-half cup vinegar, fill cup with water, one teaspoon mustard, one teaspoon flour. Cook this slowly, then pour over two well-beaten eggs, put back on stove and simmer, not boil, when cool add one-half cup cream. Garnish with rings of hard-boiled eggs.—*Mrs. C. O. Hoyt.*

Sweetbread Salad.—Soak the sweetbreads in salt and water for fifteen minutes, cover with boiling water and simmer for twenty-eight minutes. Drain, cover with cold water. As soon as cool enough to handle remove all skin and pick in pieces. For each pair of sweetbreads one-half cup of "mayonnaise" dressing will be required. Celery cut in pieces as for chicken salad, mixed with the sweetbreads. Serve on lettuce leaves or garnish with celery tops.—*Mrs. G. C. Greene.*

Apple Salad.—Take sour apples, chopped not too fine; celery chopped fine; dress with one egg well-beaten, thickened with oil drop by drop, then thinned with vinegar; add a pinch of salt and pepper. Fresh cucumbers cut into dice add a fine flavor to potato salad.—*Mrs. E. C. Chapin.*

Salmon Salad.—This dish may be prepared from either canned or cold boiled salmon. Arrange fish in neat flakes; pour over it the following dressing. This dressing may be used for lettuce alone: Yolks of three hard-boiled eggs; one tablespoon of salad oil or melted butter; rub with the egg to a smooth paste; add two teaspoons each of sugar and mustard; salt and cayenne to taste; add a little vinegar. Arrange lettuce leaves around the plate; pour the dressing on the fish and garnish with the whites of the eggs cut in rings.

Cabbage Salad.—Chop cabbage and small piece of onion fine, pour on salad dressing while hot, and mix thoroughly.

Dressing for same: Yolks of four eggs, three tablespoonfuls sugar, one teaspoonful salt, one saltspoonful red pepper, two teaspoonfuls mustard, two tablespoonfuls butter, two tablespoonfuls cream, two-thirds of a cup of vinegar. Cook until thick.—*Mary M. Robson.*

Oyster Salad.—Put two dozen small oysters in enough boiling water to cover them. Cook a few minutes until the edges begin to curl. Add a little salt and a tablespoon vinegar; drain and cool. Arrange the leaves of two heads of lettuce, place the oysters in the center, pour over them a mayonnaise sauce.—*Mrs. E. H. Whitney.*

CHICKEN SALAD.—Boil one chicken and pick up fine and cut two heads of celery fine. Dressing: Yolks of two eggs beaten; piece of butter size of an egg; melt the butter in a cup of vinegar; beat the eggs and stir the vinegar in them; set on the stove and boil, stirring all the time; sugar and salt to taste.; one teaspoonful of cornstarch stirred in and then let it get cold. After all is put together pour over one cup of sweet cream.—*Mrs. W. S. Griswold.*

SALAD DRESSING.—Mix three tablespoons of sugar; one teaspoon mustard; one teaspoon of salt together. In another dish take yolks of three eggs, beat and add two-thirds cup of vinegar. Put all in a bowl and let thicken (not boil) in the top of teakettle of boiling water; when done, add a lump of butter size of a walnut, and three tablespoons sweet cream.—*Mrs. J. J. Baird.*

CHICKEN SALAD.—Two cups of celery to one of meat. Dressing: One pint of vinegar; yolks of eight eggs; heaping teaspoon of mustard; same of salt; pinch of red pepper; one-half teacup of butter. Put the butter and vinegar on the stove, and when it boils pour it gradually on the mustard, salt, pepper, whip the eggs thoroughly and stir in; when cold add a teacup of thick cream whipped stiff.—*Mrs. John Rork.*

POTATO SALAD.—Eight large, cold, boiled potatoes, sliced rather thin; one good-sized cucumber (when cucumbers are out of season use two small pickles); four olives cut fine; three small onions sliced very thin, or chopped fine; one-half cup capers; the broken meats of seven English walnuts. Mix with plenty of mayonnaise dressing. For those who dislike oil in salad dressing I give the following recipe: One small cup vinegar; yolks of four eggs; one tablespoon butter; one of sugar; one teaspoon of mustard; a pinch of cayenne pepper; saltspoon salt. Beat yolks in a bowl with the other ingredients except butter and vinegar. Put butter in vinegar and heat quickly. When boiling hot pour over the beaten eggs, etc. Put it in a saucepan now and return to the fire. Stir constantly until thick and smooth. When cold add one-half cup of cream.—*Mrs. E. Cahill.*

POTATO SALAD.—One egg well-beaten, one-fourth of a cup of vinegar if strong, if not, one-half a cup filled up with cold water; one-half teaspoonful of salt, a little pepper, butter size of a walnut, one-half teaspoonful of mustard in vinegar, two tablespoonfuls of sugar. Put all together and stir till the mixture boils about three minutes. Chop cold boiled potatoes quite fine and mix, a layer of potatoes with onions and celery cut fine and a little of the dressing. —*Mrs. John Rork.*

PARK HOUSE SALAD DRESSING.—One teaspoonful mixed mustard, one teaspoonful sugar, one teaspoonful salt, four yolks of eggs beaten. Mix these together, then add drop by drop one-half cup of melted butter, beating constantly; then add one-half cup vinegar, cook until thick, keep beating it so that it will be smooth. When cold and you are ready to use it, add one-half cup sweet cream and if you want it extra good, beat the cream stiff before adding it.—*Mrs. B. F. Hall.*

SALMON SALAD.—One can salmon cut in small pieces; one very small head of cabbage chopped; one dozen small pickles chopped; two hard-boiled eggs chopped. Mix the ingredients well together and pour over them a pint of scalding hot vinegar, seasoning it with salt, pepper and mustard, to suit the taste.

A PRETTY SALAD.—Arrange the leaves of curly lettuce on a plate, on this slice some cucumber, add a slice or two of onion, if the flavor is desired, also some slices of tomato and radish to give color. Serve with dressing.

Chicken Salad.—Take an equal amount of cut celery and cut chicken, yolks of six eggs, one tablespoonful of mustard, one teaspoon of salt, lump of butter the size of an egg, three-quarters of a cup of vinegar, a dash of red pepper. If thick cream is added to the dressing it improves it very much. Boil until it thickens.—*Mrs. S. L. Kilbourne.*

Oyster Salad.—Let one quart of oysters come to a boil in their own liquor, then take them out, and cut or chop a little, but not fine. Add three tablespoonfuls of vinegar, one of oil, one-half teaspoonful of salt, one-half teaspoonful of pepper, and two tablespoonfuls of lemon juice. When perfectly cold, add one and one-half pints of celery, or nice white cabbage, one pint of rolled crackers, and one small cup of mayonnaise dressing or Durkee's salad dressing, with one cup of whipped cream. Use lettuce or celery leaves to garnish.—*Mrs. N. B. Jones.*

Oyster Salad.—Drain the liquor from a quart of fresh oysters. Put them in hot vinegar enough to cover them placed over the fire: let them remain until plump, but not cooked; then drop immediately into cold water, drain off and mix with them two pickled cucumbers cut fine; also a quart of celery cut in dice pieces; some seasoning of salt and pepper. Mix all well together, tossing up with a silver fork. Pour over the whole a mayonnaise dressing. Garnish with celery tips and hard-boiled eggs.

Bean Salad.—String young beans; break into half-inch pieces or leave whole; wash and cook soft in salt water; drain well; add finely-chopped onions, pepper, salt and vinegar; when cool add olive oil, melted butter or mayonnaise dressing if vinegar is left out.

EGG SALAD.—Take as many eggs as needed, boil them until perfectly hard, almost half an hour. Take out the yolks carefully, chop the white very fine. Arrange lettuce leaves or cress on a dish, making nests of the whites of eggs, and put one yolk in each nest; add a dressing made as follows: One saltspoon of salt; one-half saltspoon of pepper; three tablespoonfuls of oil; one-fourth teaspoonful of lemon juice; one tablespoonful of vinegar. Mix in the order given, adding oil slowly.—*Mrs. N. B. Jones.*

POTATO SALAD.—Take half a dozen good-sized cold potatoes and slice thin in a dish, sprinkling occasionally with salt, pepper and a cold hard-boiled egg sliced thin. When done pour in vinegar enough to cover the salad, being careful not to wash off the seasoning. Let this stand a couple of hours and then pour off the vinegar. This makes a good tea dish for warm weather. A small raw onion sliced very thin may be added if desired.—*Mrs. G. L. Freeman.*

DANDELION SALAD.—One pint of the plants carefully washed and placed in a salad bowl with an equal quantity of water-cresses, three green onions, a teaspoonful of salt and plenty of oil or cream dressing. This is one of the most healthful and refreshing of all early salads. —*Juliet Corson, N. Y.*

CORN SALAD.—Four ears of green corn, two heads of celery, four hard-boiled eggs. Boil the corn, when cold cut from cob, and scrape the cob. Cut celery and eggs in dice. Take three tablespoonfuls of cream whipped stiff, add to this four tablespoonfuls of mayonnaise dressing. Pour over salad and mix thoroughly.—*Mrs. H. R. Pratt.*

VEGETABLES.

"Society expects every man to have certain things in his garden. Not to raise cabbage, is as if one had no pew in church."

SUGGESTIONS.—Most vegetables, when peeled, are better when laid in cold water a short time before cooking. When partly cooked a little salt should be thrown in the water in which they are boiled, and they should cook steadily after they are put on, not allowed to stop simmering or boiling until done.

Onions, cabbage, carrots and turnips should be cooked in a great deal of water, and boiled only long enough to sufficiently cook them, and immediately drained.

The most nutritious part of the potato is next to the skin, therefore it should be pared thinly.

Baked potatoes are universally acceptable with cold meats for dinner, with beefsteak or picked up codfish for breakfast. They are especially good with fresh fish, fried or scalloped oysters. Never serve baked potatoes without pricking or cracking the skins to let the steam escape. Cover only with a napkin. Mashed or plain boiled potatoes should be served with stewed chicken, or roasts with which gravies are served. Turnips and cabbages seem most at home with mutton or corned beef. Sour baked apples are nice with hash for breakfast.

LYONNAISE POTATOES.—Take eight or ten good-sized cold boiled potatoes, slice them endwise, then crosswise, making them like dice in small squares. When you are ready to cook them, heat some butter or good drippings in a frying pan; fry in it one small onion (chopped fine) until it begins to change color and look yellow. Now put in your potatoes, sprinkle well with salt and pepper, stir well and cook about five minutes, taking care that you do not break them. They must not brown. Just before taking up, stir in a tablespoonful of minced parsley. Drain dry by shaking in a heated colander. Serve very hot.—*White House Cook Book.*

TOASTED POTATOES.—Slice cold boiled potatoes one-fourth of an inch thick lengthwise of the potato; place on a broiler over clear coals and toast both sides brown; dip each slice in melted butter, season with salt and pepper and place in a hot dish. When all are done pour the butter that is left over them. Serve hot, but do not cover them, as steaming spoils them. Good for breakfast or tea.—*Mrs. Clarence Bement.*

POTATO PUFF.—Take two cupfuls of cold mashed potato and stir into it two tablespoonfuls of melted butter, beating to a white cream before adding anything else. Then put with this two eggs whipped very light and a teacupful of cream or milk, salting to taste. Beat all well, pour into a deep dish and bake in a quick oven until nicely browned. If well mixed it will come out light and delectable. —*Kate T. Cooley.*

POTATO BALLS.—Take mashed potatoes, seasoned with salt and butter, make up into balls, dip into well-beaten eggs and then into bread crumbs and fry in butter a nice brown.

POTATO FILLETS.—Pare and slice the potatoes lengthwise; cut them if you like in small fillets, about a quarter of an inch square, and as long as the potato will admit; keep them in cold water until wanted, then drop them into boiling lard; when nearly done take them out with a skimmer and drain them, boil up the lard again, drop the potatoes back and fry until done; this causes the fillets to swell up and puff.—*Mrs. N. B. Jones.*

BAKED TOMATOES.—Select tomatoes of the same size, wash and remove the cores, sprinkle a little salt and pepper over them, place a small piece of butter in the centers and fill with dry bread crumbs or rolled crackers, again placing a small piece of butter on top. Put the tomatoes in a baking dish and bake in a slow oven two hours and serve hot.

SCALLOPED, OR BAKED CORN.—Take a bake tin, cover bottom with corn cut from cob or canned, then a layer of bread crumbs, a little butter, salt and pepper, then a layer of corn, etc., until the dish is nearly full, then fill with milk and bake one hour.

MOCK OYSTERS.—Six nice plump ears of sweet corn uncooked; grate from the cob; beat one egg, stirring into it flour and milk of each one tablespoonful, season with a little salt and pepper. Put about a teaspoon of butter into a suitable pan for frying, having mixed in the corn also, drop the mixture into the hot butter, one spoon in a place, turning them so as to fry brown. Serve hot for breakfast.—*Mrs. N. B. Jones.*

GREEN CORN FRITTERS.—Two cups of grated corn, two eggs, one cup of milk, a pinch of soda or baking powder, salt, one teaspoon of melted butter, flour for thin batter; stir and fry same as griddle cakes.

SCALLOPED ONIONS.—Take eight or ten onions of good size, slice them, and boil until tender. Lay them in a baking dish, put in bread crumbs, butter in small bits, pepper and salt, between each layer until the dish is full, putting bread crumbs last; add milk or cream until full. Bake 20 or 30 minutes.—*White House Cook Book.*

LADIES' CABBAGE.—Boil a firm white cabbage fifteen minutes, changing the water then for more from the teakettle. When tender, drain and set aside until perfectly cold. Chop fine and add two beaten eggs, a tablespoonful of butter, pepper, salt, three tablespoonfuls of rich milk or cream. Stir all well together, and bake in a buttered pudding dish until brown. Serve very hot. This dish is digestible and palatable, resembling cauliflower.

Stewed Cabbage.—Cut the cabbage in quarters, and wash very thoroughly in cold water, then boil in salted water until tender, drain and cover with drawn butter or cream sauce.—*Mrs. N. B. Jones.*

Baked Beets.—Beets retain their sugary delicate flavor to perfection if they are baked instead of boiled. Turn them frequently while in the oven, using a knife. as the fork allows the juices to run out. When done remove the skin and serve with butter, salt and pepper on the slices.

Asparagus with Eggs.—Boil a bunch of asparagus twenty minutes; cut off the tender tops and lay them in a deep pie plate, buttering, salting and peppering well. Beat up four eggs, the yolks and whites separately, to a stiff froth; add two tablespoonfuls of milk or cream, a tablespoonful of warm butter, pepper and salt to taste. Pour evenly over the asparagus mixture. Bake eight minutes, or until the eggs are set. Very good.

Asparagus Omelet.—Boil some tender fresh-cut asparagus in very little water with a small portion of salt, or, what is better still, steam the asparagus without water until it is tender; chop it it very fine, mix it with the yolks of five and the whites of three well-beaten eggs; add two tablespoonfuls of sweet cream; fry, serve quite hot.

Turnips a la Poulette.—Cut the turnips in dice and put in a saucepan, when boiled tender turn them into a colander. Put a little butter and flour in a saucepan and stir. Add a gill of milk and stir, then the turnips, and salt and pepper to taste.

Baked Egg Plant.—Cut into slices one-half inch thick. Sprinkle sparingly with salt and press over night. Pile the slices and turn a plate over them with a weight placed upon it. (This is to express the juice which is disagreeable to the taste.) Dip the slices into egg and then in crumbs. Have in the pan enough hot fat to prevent sticking and place in the oven till done. Another way is to fry in butter without crumbs. —*Mrs. H. B. Baker.*

Tomatoes Au Gratin.—This simple and delicious dish is made by cutting some ripe tomatoes in half, putting them in a buttered dish with breadcrumbs, butter, pepper and salt, and baking till slightly browned on top.—*The Universal Cookery Book.*

Parsnip Fritters.—Boil four or five parsnips; when tender take off the skin and mash them fine; add to them a teaspoonful of wheat flour and a beaten egg. Put a tablespoonful of lard or beef dripping in a frying pan over the fire, add to it a saltspoonful of salt; when boiling hot put in the parsnips, making them in small cakes with a spoon; when both are done take them on a dish, put a very little of the fat in which they were fried over and serve hot. These resemble the taste of salsify.—*Everyday Cook-Book.*

Stewed Celery.—Cut in inch pieces, simmer until tender in a little water, add sweet cream, sweeten to taste, and serve; or pour over slices of toasted bread and serve hot.

Baked Turnips—Wash, pare, boil one-half hour, cut in thin slices, lay in a buttered pudding dish, sprinkle with seasoned bread crumbs, moisten with milk and bake in the oven until a rich brown.

Time Table.—Giving the approximate length of time required for cooking different vegetables.

Thirty minutes.—Asparagus, corn, macaroni, mushrooms, peas, boiled potatoes, tomatoes.

Forty-five minutes.—Young beets, parsnips, turnips, baked potatoes, rice.

One hour.—New cabbage, string beans, cauliflower, greens, salsify, new onions, winter squash.

Two hours.—Carrots, parsnips, turnips and onions.

SIDE DISHES.

"The cultivated stomach appreciates contrast and harmonies in taste."

MACARONI WITH CHEESE.—Boil the macaroni about twenty minutes, then arrange alternate layers of the macaroni and cheese, grated if old, in bits if new; pour over enough milk to cover. Season to taste, and bake about twenty minutes.—*Mrs. E. H. Whitney.*

CHEESE FONDU.—Soak one cup of very dry bread crumbs in two scant cups of new milk. Beat into this three eggs whipped very light, add one small teaspoon of melted butter. Pepper and salt to taste. Lastly one cup of dry old cheese, finely grated. Butter a baking dish. pour the fondu into it. Strew dry bread crumbs over the top and bake in a quick oven to a delicate brown. Serve it immediately in the baking dish. Delicious.—*Lizzie B. Cowles.*

CHEESE STICKS —One cup grated cheese, one cup flour, a small pinch cayenne pepper, one-half cup butter; mix with cold water, roll thin, cut in strips and bake a light brown.

SCALLOPED CHEESE —Take three slices of bread, well buttered, first cutting off the brown outside crust. Grate fine a quarter of a pound of any kind of good cheese; lay the bread in layers in a buttered baking dish, sprinkle over it the grated cheese, some salt and pepper to taste. Mix four well-beaten eggs with three cups of milk; pour it over the bread and cheese. Bake it in a hot oven as you would cook a bread pudding. This makes an ample dish for four people.—*White House Cook Book.*

CHEESE CAKES.—Mix equal parts of flour, butter and grated cheese with the yolk of one egg. Season with salt and pepper. Take out on the kneading board and work in all the extra flour it will hold so it can be rolled very thin. Cut with small cutter and bake seven minutes in quick oven.—*Kate T. Cooley.*

MACARONI.—Break up in small pieces two cupfuls of the best macaroni. Put in boiling water with a little salt, cook until tender, then drain off the water and put a layer in the bottom of a baking dish, sprinkling a little salt, good generous pieces of butter and a tablespoonful of finely-grated cheese, and so on to the top, then cover it closely (after pouring over a large cupful of cream) bake covered until it seems of a jelly-like consistency, then uncover and let brown.—*Mrs. T. E. Potter.*

MACARONI WITH CHEESE.—Break one-fourth of a pound into small pieces, wash quickly in cold water, cook in boiling water one-half hour, when half done add salt, when done, drain. Butter a pudding dish, put in the macaroni and pour over it a sauce made of two tablespoons of butter warmed, stir in tablespoon flour, a little salt and pepper and one pint of cold milk, heat gradually and let it come to a boil. Put one cup grated cheese mixed with one cup fine bread crumbs over the top and bake in a quick oven fifteen or twenty minutes.—*Mrs. Clarence Bement.*

WELSH RAREBIT.—Toast bread quickly, without allowing it to dry; cut off the crust smoothly with a sharp knife, butter it and cover with thin slices of cheese, spread very lightly with made mustard, lay on a pie plate and set in the oven till melted. Cut in halves or thirds. Serve immediately.—*Mrs. J. M. Earle.*

CHESTNUT CROQUETTE.—Boil fifty sound chestnuts; take them from the shells, pound them into crumbs, rub in one ounce of butter then mix in a small cup of sweet cream, two ounces of butter and one ounce of powdered sugar, put the whole into a double boiler and stir in the beaten yolks of six eggs. Set the mixture to cool. Make into balls, dip in cracker meal and then into yolk of eggs, drop into hot lard and brown a pale yellow. If you desire then roll in sifted sugar.—*Carrie Jones.*

Fried Bananas.—Select medium-sized or small bananas, peel and dip the whole banana in beaten egg, roll in fine bread or cracker crumbs and fry in butter to a delicate brown. Sprinkle with powdered sugar and serve hot. Served on small plates and dressed with parsely they make a pretty course for a lunch.—*Mrs. Clarence Bement.*

Baked Dressing.—One quart of dry pieces of bread, one pint of milk or cold water. If you have some bits of meat, chop fine; also one small onion, then add a little sage, pepper and salt, a small piece of butter and one egg. Mix well and place in your baking dish and bake one hour. Serve hot. This is an economical dish and very good.

Rice Croquettes.—One pint of boiled rice; add yolks of two eggs, a pinch of salt; make this into balls, roll in cracker crumbs, and fry in hot lard.—*Mrs. E. E. Bush.*

Sandwiches.—One-half pound butter, two tablespoonfuls mixed mustard, two teaspoonfuls of salad oil, yolk of one egg; white pepper and salt to taste. Beat all together to a smooth paste, and place on ice to cool. Chop tongue and ham very fine, using two parts of tongue to one of ham. Spread the bread with the dressing, then with the meat.

Fritters.—One quart of Voigt's Royal patent flour, one pint of sweet milk, two teaspoons of Queen Flake baking powder, two eggs, whites and yolks beaten separately and added last, a pinch of salt. Drop from a large spoon into hot lard and fry. Eaten with maple syrup.

Sweetbreads.—Blanch these by pouring cold water on and putting them on the stove and letting them simmer for one-half hour; take them out and put in cold water, season and roll in flour and fry a light brown in lard. or butter if preferred.

To Cook Frogs' Legs.—Season with salt and pepper, some corn meal, wipe dry the frogs' legs and roll in the prepared corn meal; fry in deep lard until a delicate brown. Serve on garnished platter.

Welsh Rarebit.—Grate dry cheese, place in saucepan with just enough milk to moisten well, when hot and a smooth paste spread on squares of nicely-toasted bread; set in the oven to brown over the top. Serve very hot.—*Mrs. N. B. Jones.*

Mock Macaroni.—Take boiled rice instead of macaroni, place a layer in a baking dish, then a layer of grated cheese, butter, pepper and salt alternately, until dish is full; pour over all enough milk to cover well. Bake about thirty minutes.

Slip.—Slip is bonny clabber without its acidity, and so delicate is its flavor that many persons like it just as well as ice cream. It is thus prepared: Make a quart of milk moderately warm; then stir into it one large spoonful of the preparation called rennet; set it by and when cool again it will be as stiff as jelly. It should be made only a few hours before it is to be used, or it will be tough and watery, in summer set the dish on ice after it has jellied. It must be served with powdered sugar, nutmeg and cream.—*White House Cook Book.*

Orange Hash.—Oranges, bananas, lemons, raisins and pineapples, these fruits are minced into little bits and served with sugar and nutmeg. Eat from cups made of the orange, cut hole in the orange big enough to insert spoon, scoop out all the pulp and fill rind with hash.

Fruit Salad.—Soak three-fourths box of gelatine in cold water one hour, add two cups of boiling water, juice of four lemons and two cups of sugar; strain and mix into it six bananas, six oranges cut fine, and add a few malaga grapes cut in half and candied cherries as desired. Set in cold place, stir occasionally until it begins to harden. This makes about three pints.—*Mrs. N. B. Jones.*

Salted Peanuts.—Take unroasted peanuts, pour hot water over them and let stand on the stove until they come to a boil, remove the skins, then place on a tin with a small piece of butter and let remain in the oven until a light brown, stirring often; remove and salt.

Salted Almonds.—Blanch paper shell almonds, when dry drop in boiling butter, stir all the time; take out when light brown in skimmer, drain on blotting paper, salt well.—*Mrs. E. C. Chapin.*

EGGS.

"There is always a best way of doing everything, if it be to boil an egg."

Frothed Eggs.—Take the yolks of eight eggs and the whites of four and beat them up with a tablespoonful of water and the strained juice of one lemon. Sweeten to taste, add a pinch of salt, then fry the same as an omelet. Have ready the four remaining whites whipped to a stiff froth with a pound of pulverized sugar, and flavored with vanilla or lemon. Then dish the omelet, heap the frothed egg high upon it and put in the oven for a few minutes to brown.

Dressed Eggs.—Boil the eggs hard. When cold, halve them and remove the yolks. Mash the yolks very fine and mix with chopped celery and salad dressing. This will be found to give better satisfaction than when using meats for filling

Baked Eggs.—Mix chopped ham and bread crumbs in equal parts; season with salt and pepper and moisten with milk and melted butter. Fill gem pans half full of this batter, break an egg on top of each and sprinkle with rolled crackers and bake until the whites set. Serve hot. —*Mrs. J. H. Underhill.*

Another.—Break eight eggs into a well-buttered dish; put in pepper and salt, bits of butter, and add three tablespoonfuls of cream; set in oven and bake about twenty minutes. Serve very hot.

Scrambled Eggs.—Heat one cup of sweet milk, then rub a tablespoonful of butter with a teaspoonful of flour and stir into the boiling milk. Into this put six beaten eggs.—*Mrs. F. B. Lee.*

Omelet—Allow one egg to each person; to each egg allow five tablespoonfuls milk, one tablespoonful flour, one-third teaspoonful baking powder; salt to taste. Bake slowly for twenty minutes.—*Mary M. Robson.*

Omelet.—One cup of bread crumbs soaked, one cup of sweet milk, five eggs, whites and yolks beaten separately, salt and pepper. Bake in a hot spider.—*Mrs. H. R. Pratt.*

Omelet.—Four eggs, yolks and whites beaten separately, one-half cup sweet milk, one small tablespoon flour, a little salt; add whites the last thing, not stirring them very thoroughly through the mixture, cook slowly in a spider for about ten minutes. Cover for the first five minutes, then lift from the center lightly and carefully with a fork to prevent sticking. Repeat this three or four times until cooked.—*Mrs. N. B. Jones.*

Creamed Eggs.—Six eggs boiled half an hour, lay in cold water until quite cold. Six slices of toast on a hot platter, one-half pint cream sauce. Put a layer of sauce on each slice of toast, part of the white of the eggs cut in rings; rub part of the yolks through a sieve over it. Repeat. Finish with a third layer of sauce, and place in the oven a few moments. Garnish with parsley.

CREAM SAUCE.—One pint of milk or cream, one heaping tablespoonful of flour, salt and pepper to suit. Let the cream come to a boil, and stir in the butter and flour rubbed to a cream. Boil up once. If milk is used a large tablespoonful of butter should be used.

OMELET.—Five eggs, beaten separately, one scant teacup of milk, one tablespoonful of flour mixed smooth with a little milk, salt and pepper to taste. Beat the whites stiff and add the last thing. Have an iron spider hot and well covered with butter, pour in half of the omelet. When brown on the bottom set in the oven a few moments. When done fold and serve at once. Chopped ham or grated cheese may be sprinkled over it before folding together. Should be made as quickly as possible, as it spoils to stand either before or after cooking.—*Mrs. W. K. Prudden.*

ESCALLOPED EGGS.—Four or eight hard-boiled eggs, one-half cup of butter. two cupfuls of rolled crackers, one stalk of celery chopped fine. Cut the eggs lengthwise, placing in an earthen dish in layers, crumbs and eggs, seasoned with salt and pepper and the chopped celery and bits of butter. Pour over all milk enough to soften, and bake in a hot oven twenty minutes. Serve with olives or cut pickles sprinkled over crust.

SCRAMBLED EGGS AND OYSTERS.—Beat the eggs together, add a little cream, chop the oysters well, salt and pepper to taste, scramble all together. Serve on slices of buttered toast.

A DAINTY WAY FOR PREPARING EGGS.—Take as many eggs as you wish to cook; separate whites from yolks, leaving yolks whole, beat whites very stiff and arrange in the form of little nests on a greased platter (or individual dishes), place one yolk in each nest, put into hot oven and brown. Serve immediately and season on table.—*Mrs. Chester Brown, Lake Charles, La.*

Fresh eggs sink when when put into a basin of cold water, the stale will rise and float. If the large end turns up in the water they are not fresh.

BREAD.

"A simple meal of bread and butter is a feast when beautified by the graces of good breeding."

SUGGESTIONS.

Much less time is required for kneading dough made from choice than from inferior brands of flour. It is economy of time and material to buy the best.

Perfect success cannot be obtained in bread making if the ferment or sponge is allowed to change temperature, alternating from cold to heat, seventy-five to eighty degrees steadily maintained yielding the best results. A heavy earthen bowl is better than wood or tin for mixing, and the dough should be well covered to protect from draughts. "The true housewife makes her bread the sovereign of her kitchen, its behests must be attended to in all critical points, no matter what else is postponed. In the earlier stages of bread making there is no danger of working the bread too much, but after all the flour is in, and has been well worked and perfectly fermented, the less it is manipulated the better. In baking, the oven should be hot enough to brown a teaspoonful of flour in five minutes, and the heat should be greater at the bottom than at the top of the oven.

"Always bake small, thin loaves, unless forced to economize oven-room, as they are sweeter than large ones. Graham bread does not require so hot an oven as white bread but should bake long. Try baking first and steaming after for recipes which call for steaming followed by baking."

Champion Yeast.—At breakfast time take three heaping tablespoonfuls of flour, two level tablespoonfuls of sugar, two level tablespoonfuls of salt. Put these into a bowl and pour on one pint of *boiling* water stirring all the time. When luke warm stir in two yeast cakes, which have been previously dissolved in one cup of luke-warm water. Set this in a warm place until noon, then pare twelve medium-sized potatoes, boil them in three pints of water. When done put through a colander—or a vegetable sieve is better—and add one quart of cold water. When luke warm add the yeast mixture and set in a warm place till morning.

One quart of this will make four loaves. I divide the yeast equally and put into four quart cans. The cans will not be full but the yeast sometimes rises and fills the cans. Stand away in a cool place—not too cool—and use for bread as follows:

THE CHAMPION BREAD.—Take one can of the yeast and if not full fill with luke-warm water; add to it one tablespoon of melted lard and one teaspoon of salt. Stir in flour until thick enough to knead. Work one-half hour and put back in the dish for a second rising. When light mold quickly and lightly into small loaves, put in the baking tins and set in a warm place for one-half hour. Bake until the loaves are loose in the pans. Prick the loaves with a fork before baking and rub lightly with melted butter, or any clean, sweet lard or fryings. If the dish in which bread is set to rise is greased before putting the dough in, it will not stick to the dish when taken out to mold, and thus prevent both waste of time and material.—*Mrs. A. O. Bement.*

Excellent results are obtained from the foregoing receipt by omitting the teaspoonful of salt and stirring into the quantity of yeast indicated flour to make a batter a trifle thicker than for griddle cakes and beating thirty minutes with paddle or wooden spoon. Then add flour enough to mould into loaves, knead thoroughly and place in warm pans to rise for one or two hours, according to season of year. The beating at the early stage of the process gives a fine grain and tenderness of texture, and is easier for many than the long-continued kneading.—*Mrs. N. B. Jones.*

SALT RISING BREAD.—Pour half a pint of boiling water on two

tablespoonfuls of corn meal and a pinch of salt. When cool stir in two tablespoonfuls of flour and set in a warm place to rise over night. In the morning add half a pint of warm water and flour enough to make the yeast smooth. Put this in a kettle of warm water until light, being careful not to let the water get too warm When this rises, pour it into a batter made of two quarts of scalded milk, when cooled, add flour. Beat this well and set to rise in a warm place. Now stir in flour to make a stiff batter that cannot be stirred with a spoon, turn out on the moulding board, mould into this a piece of lard the size of a small apple make into loaves and when light bake as soon as possible, as the bread will be much whiter and better. Care must be taken not to scald the yeast, rising or dough.—*Mrs. J. F. Dublin.*

Corn Bread.—One cup corn meal, one cup Royal patent flour, two-thirds cup molasses, two-thirds teaspoon soda, a little salt, water to make medium batter. This will be enough to fill half full two well-greased baking powder cans. Put on cover to steam two hours. Bake half an hour. Let stand a few minutes before taking off cover; turn bottom side up.—*Mrs. W. Donovan.*

Graham Bread.—Two cups buttermilk, one-third of shortening, one-third of molasses, one teaspoonful soda, salt, one-third flour, two-thirds graham. Mix very thick with spoon. After baked, wrap in a damp cloth.—*Mrs. A. J. Lamphere.*

Boston Brown Bread.—Two cups of sour milk, two tablespoonfuls sugar, one rounded teaspoonful soda, one scant half cup of molasses, one teaspoonful salt, one half cup of corn meal, then thicken with graham flour or Voigt's Flouroigt until it stirs stiff with a spoon. Melt a piece of lard as large as a walnut in your baking tin (I use a small deep bread pan) then put mixture in and bake one hour in a very slow oven. This is excellent.—*Mrs. C. C. Wood.*

One Loaf Graham Bread.—Two and a half cups graham flour, one-third cup molasses, pinch of salt, a little melted shortening, teaspoonful soda, and sour milk enough to make a thick batter. Bake rather slow. —*Mrs. E. N. Perrin.*

Brown Bread.—One and one-half cups of buttermilk, one-half cup of molasses, two small teaspoons of soda, one teaspoon of salt. Stir stiff with graham flour. Bake in a moderate oven.—*Mrs. D. M. Hough.*

Brown Bread.—Butter size of a walnut, one large tablespoonful of brown sugar, salt, one egg, beat all until smooth, then stir in two cups of sour milk, and two cups of graham flour after which stir in one large tablespoonful of molasses, one teaspoonful of saleratus, one cup of graham flour and one-half cup of white flour. Bake in a moderate oven one hour.—*Mrs. J. B. Porter.*

Brown Bread.—One and one-half cups sour milk, one cup molasses, one well-rounded teaspoon soda, one teaspoon salt, one cup each of corn meal, rye flour and graham meal; enough for three one-pound B. P. cans. Steam two hours.—*Mrs. T. E. Potter.*

Brown Bread.—One and one-half cups sour milk, one half cup molasses, one egg, one teaspoon soda, pinch of salt, graham flour to stir quite thick. Steam two hours.—*Mrs. Chas. Broas.*

Brown Bread.—Two cups of sour milk, half cup of molasses, two eggs, one teaspoonful of soda dissolved in a little cold water, one cup of flour, two cups of graham flour; bake till brown.—*Mrs. John Whiteley.*

Brown Bread (Baked).—Into one cup warm water stir one-half cup yeast, two cups flour, one half cup molasses, one-half cup brown sugar, and a pinch of salt. Add Flouroigt flour until stiff as can be stirred with spoon. Make into loaves and let rise in tins over night. Bake in moderate oven.

Boston Brown Bread.—One cup graham flour, one cup corn meal, one-half cup wheat flour, one-half cup molasses, one teaspoon soda, one cup sweet milk. Boil in tin can, a pound baking powder can is good. Grease the can, fill with the batter, putting the cover on, set the can into a flat-bottom kettle with water enough to come nearly to the top of the can, keep boiling for three hours then remove the cover, setting the can into the oven for about five minutes.—*Viola S. Moffett.*

BOSTON BROWN BREAD.—Two cups of sweet milk, one cup of sour milk; one cup of molasses, one dessertspoon of soda, two cups of graham flour, one cup of rye flour, one cup of Indian meal, a little salt. Steam four hours then bake half an hour.

BROWN BREAD —One cup sweet milk, one cup sour milk, one cup brown sugar, two cups graham flour, one cup corn meal, teaspoon soda, and salt. Steam three hours.

GRAHAM BREAD.—One pint of bread dough, one scant cup of molasses, one egg, pinch of salt, one cup warm water. Stir in graham flour or Voigt's Flouroigt so that it will drop from a spoon. Leave in the dish until light. Then beat it and turn into a greased dish, let it rise again and bake.—*Mrs. Albert Clark.*

CORN BREAD OR INDIAN LOAF.—Soak bits of dry bread in water, say about two teacupfuls, then add two cups of sour milk, one cup of sugar, salt, two teaspoons of soda, two cups fine corn meal, half cup of Voigt's Royal Patent flour. Steam two hours then put in hot oven twenty minutes A good way to dispose of dry bread.—*Charlotte Cook Book.*

STEAMED BROWN BREAD.—One cup of white flour (Voigt's Royal Patent). two of graham flour, or Voigt's Flouroigt, two of Indian meal, one teaspoonful of soda, one cup of molasses, three and one-half cups of milk, a little salt. Beat well and steam four hours. This is for sour milk; when sweet milk is used, use Queen Flake baking powder in place of soda. This is improved by setting it into the oven fifteen minutes after it is slipped from the mould. To be eaten warm with butter. Most excellent.—*White House Cook Book.*

Boston Brown Bread.—Three cups of corn meal, three cups of rye flour, three cups of buttermilk, one cup of molasses, two scant teaspoons of soda. Steam three hours, then bake fifteen minutes.—*Miss Daly.*

Brown Bread.—One cup of brown sugar, one egg, four tablespoons of melted butter, one-half cup of sour cream, one and one-half cup of sour milk, one teaspoon soda, a little salt, graham flour enough for a soft batter.—*Miss Tillie Bodamer.*

BREAKFAST AND TEA CAKES.

Parker House Rolls.—Rub one-half tablespoon of butter and one-half tablespoon of lard into two quarts of sifted Royal patent flour; cut a well in the middle of the flour, pour one pint of cold boiled milk and add one-half cup of yeast, one-half cup of sugar and a little salt. If wanted for tea, rub the flour and butter and boil the milk and cool the night before. Add sugar, yeast and salt, and turn all into the flour, but do not stir. Let it stand over night; in the morning stir up, knead and let rise till near tea time, then mould, cut with cake cutter, put a little melted butter on one half and lap neatly over on the other half. Place in the pan about three-quarters of an inch apart and bake quickly.—*Mrs. Gertrude Barry.*

Pop-overs.—One cup of milk, two teaspoons of Queen Flake baking powder, piece of butter the size of an egg, two cups of sifted Royal patent flour, one egg, well beaten. Bake in a hot oven in gem pans. A scant tablespoon of butter will make a large pop-over if oven and gem pans are just right.—*Mrs. E. Marvin.*

MUFFINS.—Two cups sifted Royal patent flour, one-half teaspoon salt. In another bowl break two eggs, beat very light, add two-thirds cup sweet milk and two tablespoons melted butter, mix well together. Add to the flour and salt one-half teaspoon sugar, turn contents of the bowl into the flour and stir thoroughly. When all is ready add one heaping teaspoon of baking powder, bake about twenty minutes in gem pans.—*Carrie Jones.*

MOLLIE'S MUFFINS.—One egg, two tablespoons white sugar, one tablespoon lard, one cup sweet milk, two cups Voigt's Royal patent flour, one teaspoon Queen Flake baking powder, salt to taste. Try these.—*Mary Wright.*

MUFFINS.—One and one-half cups of milk, two cups of flour, one egg, a piece of butter the size of a small egg, one teaspoon sugar, one-half teaspoon salt, two full teaspoons Queen Flake baking powder. Stir the flour into the milk, beat the egg until very light, and to it add the melted butter, sugar and salt, mix with the batter, then add the baking powder and beat thoroughly.—*Mrs. Lucy C. Davis.*

OATMEAL BREAKFAST-MUFFINS.—Soak one cup rolled oatmeal over night in a cup of water; in the morning add one-half teaspoon salt, one cup Voigt's Royal patent flour, one-half cup milk and two teaspoons Queen Flake baking powder sifted in with the flour, dip into hot gem-irons and bake in a moderately quick oven.—*Mrs. Belle M. Perry, Charlotte, Mich.*

STEAMED BREAD IN CUPS.—One pint sour milk, one-half cup corn meal, one-half cup Voigt's Royal patent flour, two cups graham or Flouroigt, two-thirds cup brown sugar, one teaspoonful soda, one teaspoonful salt, one-third cup shortening. Steam two hours.

GRAHAM GEMS.—One tablespoonful of butter, two of sugar, one teaspoonful of soda dissolved in hot water; cream all together, then add two cupfuls of sour milk and two of graham flour. Bake in a hot oven.—*Mrs. Toolan.*

Granola Gems.—Into three-quarters of a cup of rick milk stir one cup of Granola add a pinch of salt and a few bits of chopped dates. Drop into heated irons and bake twenty or thirty minutes.—*Mrs. H. B. Baker.*

Bread Griddle Cakes.—Pieces of stale bread may be utilized in making delicious cakes in the following manner: Soak the bread in buttermilk over night. Into the milk in the morning beat soda, a scant teaspoon to a large cup of milk, add a saltspoon of salt, flour enough to make a rather stiff batter, and fry on a hot griddle.—*Mrs. Jessie M. Turner.*

Sweet Milk Pan-Cakes.—One pint sweet milk, a little salt. Mix with flour to make good batter, one egg well beaten, a little melted butter. Beat these into the batter a long time, then beat in one and one-half heaping teaspoons baking powder.—*Mrs. J. E. Nichols.*

Tea Rolls.—Three and one-half cupfuls sweet milk, one cup shortening (lard or butter), one cup yeast, one tablespoonful sugar, and a little salt. Stir stiff with flour and let rise over night. In the morning add one egg and mould. When this gets light make into rolls and after having become light again, bake.—*Kittie Walker.*

Corn Muffins.—One cup of Indian meal, two cups of Voigt's Royal Patent flour, two cups of sweet milk, two eggs, a little salt, two teaspoonfuls soda, four of cream tartar. Have the irons quite hot before putting in the batter.—*Mrs. H. P. Bartlett.*

A New Way of Serving Toast.—Take three hard-boiled eggs and when perfectly cold remove the whites and chop them fine in a chopping bowl. Toast slices of bread a delicate brown, dip very lightly into hot salted water and lay on a platter and spread butter on sparingly. Make a milk sauce as for milk toast but a little thicker. Stir into this the chopped whites of the eggs. Pour it nicely over the toast and then with a vegetable squeezer drop the yolks of the eggs prettily over the toast for decoration.—*Mrs. A. O. Bement.*

FRENCH TOAST.—Beat two eggs, add one pint milk, cut bread into thin slices, dip in the mixture and fry brown.

TO COOK OATMEAL.—Into the dish in which it is to be cooked, pour three cups of boiling water, salt to taste, stir in slowly and thoroughly one full cup of oatmeal. Cook on slow fire twenty minutes, stir only enough to keep from burning. If cooked in a farina kettle, be sure the water in outside kettle is boiling and cook not less than forty minutes.—*Mrs. J. B. Porter.*

OLDFASHIONED JOHNNYCAKE.—One cup Voigt's Royal Patent flour, one cup fine yellow corn meal, one-fourth cup sugar, one and one-half teaspoonfuls salt, two teaspoonfuls Queen Flake baking powder, one egg well beaten, one cup milk, one tablespoonful butter, softened. Mix in order given, beat well, pour into a well-greased pan, bake in a moderate oven from twenty to twenty-five minutes.—*Mrs. F. M. Howe.*

JOHNNYCAKE.—Two cups Indian meal, one cup white flour, two even teaspoonfuls soda stirred in two cups sour milk, one egg, two teaspoonfuls sugar, three tablespoons melted butter or drippings.—*Mrs. Henry Gibbs.*

CORN MEAL GEMS.—Two cups of sour milk, two eggs, one cup corn meal, one-half cup Voigt's Royal patent flour, one tablespoonful lard, one teaspoon of soda and one of salt.—*Mrs. C. J. Hazleton, Omaha, Nebraska.*

BREAKFAST MUFFINS.—One cup sugar, one egg, one tablespoon of melted butter, one pint of sweet milk, three cups of Voigt's Royal patent flour, two teaspoons of Queen Flake baking powder, one small teaspoon of salt.—*Miss Elizabeth O'Connor.*

MUFFINS.—Two eggs well beaten, one quart sifted Voigt's Royal patent flour, two teaspoons Queen Flake baking powder, one teaspoon of butter, and one teaspoon of lard melted together and put in the last thing, milk enough to make a thick batter, bake in hot buttered gem tins.—*Mrs. Roxie Donovan.*

RICE CROQUETTES.—Boil small one-half cup of rice in one pint of milk, with a pinch of salt; when cold add one egg beaten very light, with flour enough to roll; fry in lard and sift powdered sugar over when done.—*Mrs. Emma Haskell.*

SPANISH BUNS—Four eggs, save the whites of three for frosting; two cups of sugar, three-fourths cup of butter, one cup sweet milk, two teaspoons cinnamon, two of cloves, two teaspoons of Queen Flake baking powder, two and one-half cups Voigt's Royal patent flour; bake in dripping pan.

Icing for Buns.—Whites of three eggs, one and one-half cups sugar. —*Mrs. J. H. Underhill.*

GRAHAM GEMS.—One and one-half cups sour milk, two-thirds teaspoon soda, one large spoon of sugar, two teaspoons melted butter, one egg. To the egg add the milk, then the salt and sugar, then the graham flour or Flouroigt, with the soda stirred in, to make a stiff batter, so that it it will drop from the spoon. Have the gem pans hot, grease, fill and bake in hot oven.—*Mrs. Wm. Donovan.*

JOHNNYCAKE.—Three-fourths of a cup of corn meal, one and one-half cups Voigt's Royal patent flour, one-half cup of sugar, one egg, pinch of salt, two teaspoons Queen Flake baking powder, butter the size of an egg, cup of milk. Sift meal, flour and baking powder together, then add other ingredients.—*Mrs. Emma Haskell.*

TEA CAKES.—One-half cup of butter, one cup sugar, one egg, one-half cup water, teaspoon soda, flavor with a little cinnamon, and put in Royal patent flour enough to roll out. Cut with small cookie cutter and bake in a quick oven.—*Mrs. G. L. Freeman.*

BAKING POWDER BISCUIT.—Sift one quart of Voigt's Royal patent flour with two heaping teaspoons of Queen Flake baking powder. Rub into it one tablespoon of lard or butter until no lard or butter remains in lumps; also mix in a teaspoon of salt. Never roll less than one inch in thickness, cut with biscuit cutter and bake in quick oven ten or fifteen minutes.—*Mrs. A. D. Baughman.*

HUCKLEBERRY GEMS.—One cup of sweet milk, two cups of Voigt's Royal Patent flour, one egg, one tablespoon of sugar, one tablespoon of of butter, two teaspoons of Queen Flake baking powder. Mix one small teacup of huckleberries with one-third of a cup of flour and stir into batter. Bake in gem pans in quick oven fifteen to twenty minutes. Nice for tea.—*Mrs. N. B. Jones.*

CORN MUSH.—Put fresh water in a kettle to boil, salt to suit taste, when it boils stir in the meal letting it sift through the fingers slowly to prevent lumps, adding a little faster at the last until as thick as can be conveniently stirred with one hand; set in oven in kettle, bake one hour and it will be thoroughly cooked. A delicious breakfast dish is made by slicing cold mush thin and frying in a little hot lard.—*Charlotte Cook Book.*

DROP BISCUIT.—One quart of Voigt's Royal patent flour, three teaspoons of Queen Flake baking powder, tablespoonful of sugar, half a teacup of lard worked in the flour, add sweet milk enough to make a thick batter. Drop in little pans or muffin rings and bake.—*Universal Cookery Book.*

TEA ROLLS.—Take enough bread dough for one small loaf. Work into it the white of an egg, one tablespoonful of butter, and flour enough to make a firm dough. Let it stand four or five hours. Roll out an inch thick, cut out with a small biscuit cutter, fold over and place in pan about an inch apart. When light bake in a very hot oven.—*Saginaw Cook Book.*

FLANNEL ROLLS.—One quart of milk, four eggs well beaten, Royal patent flour sufficient to make a thin batter, and salt to taste. Put in cups four inches deep and bake quickly in hot oven.

SALLY LUNN.—One cup sweet milk, one-half cup butter, three cups Voigt's Royal patent flour, two tablespoons sugar, two scant tablespoonfuls Queen Flake baking powder, three eggs and a pinch of salt.

GRAHAM PUFFS.—One cup Voigt's Flouroigt or graham flour, one-half cup wheat flour, one and one-quarter cups sweet milk, one egg, one tablespoonful melted butter, and one tablespoonful Queen Flake baking powder.

BREAKFAST PUFFS.—One cup of flour, one cup of sweet milk, one tablespoonful of melted butter, one egg and a pinch of salt. Fill muffin cups about half full and bake in a quick oven.

DIET FOR THE SICK.

BY HELEN CAMPBELL, PROFESSOR OF HOUSEHOLD ECONOMICS, MADISON UNIVERSITY.

The doctors of even a generation ago had but dim comprehension of the place of food in accomplishing a cure, but each year sees more and more stress laid upon it. Within the past year or two the students of the New York Medical College have been required to take a course of sick cookery, such as is given to trained nurses, and soon every graduating medical student will be made to think it as essential a part of his work as his anatomy or chemistry. Treatises on food are increasing in number and on all sides the bearing of food on health is receiving an attention never given before.

For the ordinary reader there are two which cover the necessary ground very thoroughly: "Sick Cookery," by Miss Mary Boland, a trained nurse of wide experience, and "Diet for the Sick,"* by Mrs. Mary F. Henderson, who prepared the manual under the careful supervision of two physicians. Dietaries for different diseases are given, a series of bills of fare for convalescents, and every form of food allowed in sickness. Drinks and broths have large space, and the book is a necessity in every family, since sickness is something all must deal with at one time or another.

In the space at our command only a few dishes can be given, with the addition of two or three bills of fare, these being intended for convalescents requiring simple but very nutritious food. In preparing and serving food for any invalid, the most delicate cleanliness is necessary.

Spotless napkins, shining glass and silver, and care to prevent slopping over as one carries the tray, are the right of every invalid, and appetite will often be absolutely destroyed where they are lacking. The best broth or gruel in a thick stone china cup or plate will perhaps be rejected when a poorer thing served in delicate china will be eaten with enjoyment. Careful service is a large factor in quick recovery, and it is now part of a nurse's business to study the most perfect method both of preparation and serving.

Prepare only a small amount of anything, and never discuss it beforehand. A surprise will often arose a flagging appetite. Remember that chemistry has proven that gelatine is not nourishing, and do not be satisfied to feed a patient on jellies. Bread from any brown flour will be more nourishing than the ordinary wheat flour. Corn meal is especially valuable for thin, chilly invalids, as it contains so much heat. A wooden tray, with legs six or seven inches high, is very convenient for serving meals.

Breakfast.—A mould of cracked wheat or germea made in a cup and turned out with cream about it. Sippets of thin, lightly-buttered toast. A cup of boiling hot water with sugar and cream. Better than tea or coffee.

Dinner.—A slice of rare roast beef, or piece of broiled beefsteak, a baked potato, apple sauce, a chocolate custard.

Supper.—A rice cone with hot sauce, graham bread and a glass of grape juice.

Breakfast.—A slice of Boston brown bread hot with cream. poached egg on thin toast, hot water and cream.

Dinner.—Fricasseed chicken and mashed potato, a little lettuce or endive dressed with the gravy of the fricassee and a few drops of lemon juice, whole wheat flour pudding, hot sauce.

Supper.—A samall dish of spaghetti and tomato sauce, stewed peaches, dry toast thin, and hot water and cream.

Breakfast.—Oatmeal porridge, oysters on toast, a cup of cocoa or chocolate.

Dinner.—A lamb or mutton chop with baked potato, spinach on toast, a baked custard.

Supper.—Corn meal mush and milk.

Breakfast.—A sweetbread with rice and cream sauce, a cup of Alkethrepta and dry toast.

Dinner.—Broiled chicken and stewed corn, farina pudding.

Supper.—Hard whole wheat rolls and grape juice.

Breakfast.—Boiled eggs, baked apple and cream, corn bread.

Dinner.—A breast of prairie chicken or game, mashed potatoes, stewed tomatoes, corn flour cottage pudding.

Supper.—Wheat germ porridge and cream.

Breakfast.—Raw egg whipped, thin, buttered toast, sweet oranges sliced.

Dinner.—Cup of clear soup, stewed chicken with rice, cauliflower with cream sauce, lemon jelly.

Supper.—Granulated wheat pudding, stewed prunes with cream, a cup of cocoa.

BEEF TEA.—The old method of making beef tea by boiling the minced beef, as was often done, putting it in a bottle and so extracting the juice, gave as a result simply a stimulant, only that property of the meat remaining. Unless eggs, oatmeal or some such addition is made, there is absolutely no nourishment in beef tea, and doctors no longer prescribe it as such. Beef extract is prepared as follows: Half a pound of finely minced beef, one pint of pure water, four drops of muriatic acid, half a saltspoonful of salt. Dilute the acid in three-quarters of a pint of the water, mixing well; add the salt and mix all with the meat. Let stand an hour, strain through a hair sieve and rinse the residue with the extra quarter of a pint of water. If the patient objects to the red color it can be given in a red wine glass.

Beef Tea for Convalescents.—Cut a pound of lean beef into small bits and soak for an hour in a pint of pure soft water, then cover closely and boil for ten minutes or put in the oven and let it remain for an hour. Pour off the juice, season with a saltspoonful of salt, and use, with thin toast or wafers.

Beef, Tapioca and Egg Broth.—One pound of lean beef prepared as for beef tea and soaked for an hour in a quart of cold water. Boil slowly for two hours. Strain it. Add a half teaspoonful of salt and half a cupful of tapioca which has been washed and soaked an hour in warm water. Boil slowly for half an hour. Serve in a shallow bowl in which a poached egg is put at the last, or stir a well-beaten egg into a large cupful of the boiling soup and serve at once with wafers or crackers.

Chicken Broth.—The bones and a pound of meat from a chicken put on in three pints of cold water. Skim thoroughly when it comes to a boil, add a teaspoonful of salt and simmer slowly three hours. Strain and serve. A tablespoonful of soaked rice or tapioca may be added after the broth is strained in which case it must be returned to the fire to simmer half an hour longer.

Dr. Gaunt's Rice Jelly.—Take four tablespoonfuls of rice and boil hard for twenty minutes in three pints of water; then let it simmer for two hours. Force through a fine hair strainer, and allow it to cool. Place in an ice chest over night. To use dissolve two tablespoonfuls of it in half a pint of milk. Very useful in intestinal troubles

Indian or Corn Meal Gruel.—One quart of boiling water; one teaspoonful of salt. Mix three tablespoonfuls of corn meal with a little cold water and stir in slowly. Boil one hour; strain and serve; a cupful at once.

ARROWROOT JELLY.—To make arrowroot jelly, moisten three heaping tablespoonfuls of the best Bermuda arrowroot with a little cold water and turn into a large cup of water that is boiling over the fire and in which two teaspoonfuls of granulated sugar have been dissolved. Stir until clear and add one tablespoonful of brandy or three of wine. Wet in cold water individual moulds or small cups and pour in the liquid jelly, and put in a cold place to harden. Serve with whipped cream. When wine cannot be used, in place of it take one teaspoonful of lemon juice.

TAPIOCA JELLY—Tapioca jelly is excellent. To prepare it soak one cup of tapioca in three cups of cold water over night. In the morning put it in a double boiler with a cup of hot water and let it simmer until perfectly clear, stirring often. Sweeten to taste and flavor with the juice of half a lemon and two tablespoonfuls of wine. Pour into cups and set away until perfectly cold. Whipped cream and sugar may be served with this jelly.

If preferred, a blanc mange may be made with tapioca and milk by soaking a cup of tapioca in two cups of water over night. Place over the fire in a double boiler the soaked tapioca and stir into it two generous cups of boiling milk, three tablespoonfuls of sugar, and a pinch of salt. Let it cook slowly fifteen minutes, stirring several times. Remove from the fire and flavor with wine or vanilla. Pour into individual moulds and set away to harden.

SCOTCH PANADA.—To make Scotch panada use six Boston crackers and scatter a little granulated sugar and a grain of salt over each cracker. Put them in a bowl and just cover with boiling water. Grate a little nutmeg over them and add two tablespoonfuls of wine. Cover the dish and let it stand in a warm place until the crackers are soaked, but not broken. Serve in the bowl.

Orange Jelly.—Orange jelly will often tempt, and looks inviting. To make it, soak half a package of Cox gelatine in a teacup of cold water for an hour. Select perfect oranges and cut them through the centre and remove the inside, keeping the divided orange skins whole. Take a generous half-pint of orange juice, beat the white of an egg to a stiff froth and add to the juice with a teacup of granulated sugar, a scant pint of hot water, and the soaked gelatine. Set the dish containing the mixture over a fire in a pan of boiling water and stir until it is thoroughly heated. Strain and fill the orange cups, and put in a cold place to harden.

Cream and Milk Soups.—Cream soups are a pleasing change after plain broths or teas. Sago, pearl tapioca, barley or rice may be used. Take any white stock that is rich and well seasoned. Put into a saucepan a half pint of the stock and the same quantity of cream. When it comes to a boil add one tablespoonful of flour thoroughly moistened with cold milk, and let it boil up once. Have the tapioca or whatever you wish to use in the soup cooked and add it to the soup and serve. Barley requires two hours to cook, rice one hour; sago and pearl tapioca must be soaked in cold water half an hour and cooked the same length of time.

Chicken Jelly.—Chicken jelly may be used in a variety of ways. To make the jelly, take a fowl weighing about three pounds. Clean and remove the skin and fat. Cut it into pieces and put them into a saucepan with two generous quarts of water, a bay leaf, and some pieces of celery. Cover and heat slowly up to the boiling point Let it simmer for four hours, then season with salt and strain into glasses and set away to cool. When cold remove the fat. This jelly may be used cold or heated, and served like soup. Heat a glass of the jelly and add a gill of sherry or Madeira wine, one teaspoonful of dissolved gelatine, some sugar and the juice of half a lemon. Pour the liquid jelly into small cups and set away to harden. This makes a very nourishing wine jelly.

Pieces of the white meat of the fowl may be cut fine and put into a jelly glass and the liquid jelly poured over them. When cold it is appetizing, sliced and put between thin pieces of bread, buttered, and with the crust taken off, or with slices of jellied chicken with toasted crackers.

Boiled Rice with Egg.—Boiled rice with egg is excellent and generally liked. Wash thoroughly half a cup of rice and put it into a double boiler with just enough water to cover it. When the rice is nearly done, if any water remains, pour it off and add one cup of milk and a little salt. Let the rice cook slowly until done. Beat an egg thoroughly, and the last thing before taking the rice from the fire stir the egg into it as lightly as possible and serve hot with sugar and cream.

ADDITIONAL.

BY MARIE ARRUDA, GRADUATE NURSE-TRAINING SCHOOL.

Graham Gruel or Oatmeal.—One tablespoon cream, one-half cup boiling water, pinch of salt, one teaspoon sugar, one tablespoon graham flour stirred in slowly. Boil slowly one-half hour. Strain through a fine strainer. Add two tablespoons cream. Beat well.

Toast Coffee.—Toast three slices of bread, over which pour one pint boiling water, pour off water and add one-third cup of cream.

To Prepare Steak for the Sick.—Scrape the meat and broil. Add a little salt and butter.

Barley Water for the Sick.—To half a cup of well-washed barley add two quarts of water. Boil half an hour. When cool add equal quantity of milk. Sweeten to taste.

A Drink for the Sick.—Strain the beef tea carefully and keep ice around it. Just as it is taken put a small piece of ice in it. A patient will often drink freely of this when hot beef tea would be rejected. Do not call it beef tea in this case, but broth or drink.

BEEF TEA.—Chop fine a pound of lean beef, put it in a wide-mouthed jar, stand it in a saucepan of water and boil slowly until the juice of the meat is extracted; skim and strain, if greasy, and give cold or hot.

Slightly broil a pound of lean beef. The steak from the haunch or round is best. Cut it into strips and squeeze out the juice with a lemon squeezer. Give it cold with a little salt and celery essence. A tablespoonful of claret wine may be added. A pound of meat makes about three tablespoons of juice. This is very easily assimilated and is much to be preferred to beef tea.

Put a quart of milk into a large, perfectly clean bottle, drop in the whites of three raw egg, cork it and shake hard. Give the patient as much as he will take.

Milk may in almost all cases be given with safety, and will be kept down when all other things produce nausea. In such case add to one pint of milk four tablespoons of limewater, or more if ordered, and give two wineglassfuls at a time at short intervals. Brandy can be added to this if ordered and if the patient can retain it.

To one pint of milk slightly warmed, stir in a large dessertspoon of liquid rennet and set it aside to cool. This makes a soft blanc mange very easily swallowed.

Reading aloud, or in the presence of the patient, is never admissible unless asked for, and should never be long continued. If reading aloud is agreeable to the patient, or is permitted, read in an even, rather low voice, without much emphasis and without gesture. Do not make little pauses to pick out scraps for your own reading while the patient waits, and do not fold and refold a newspaper, or rattle the leaves of a book as you turn them. Be quiet and self-possessed at all times.

How Doses of Ipecac Should be Given.—It is better to give small doses and repeat them if necessary. For this purpose about half a teaspoonful of syrup of ipecacuanha may be given to a child under a year old, and repeated in twenty minutes if no vomiting occurs. When free vomiting has been produced, one-half the quantity can be given at the same interval, so as to keep the child slightly nauseated. A child between one and two may have a half larger dose.

A moist atmosphere tends to relieve the breathing. This can be secured by keeping water boiling in the room, one tablespoon turpentine to two quarts of water.

A child subject to croup should be guarded from the changes of the weather with unusual care.

DESSERTS.

"The true cook, be it known, is an artist."

PIES, PUDDINGS, AND CREAMS.

Piecrust.—Take three cups of sifted Royal patent flour, one cup of lard and a little salt; cut, and mix with the lard through the flour with a knife, then one-half cup of cold water, still stirring with the knife; mix as little as possible after the water has been added and do not handle more than absolutely necessary.—*Charlotte Cook-book.*

Pastry.—One-half cup butter, one-half cup lard, one pint Royal patent flour, whip in ice water with a fork. Better to let it stand awhile. Handle as little as possible.—*Mrs. C. J. Davis.*

Pie Crust.—Half pound lard, one pound Voigt's Royal patent flour, rub well together; use ice water enough to wet the lard and flour, a pinch of salt; mix it lightly.—*Mrs. F. Lutz.*

MOCK MINCE PIE.—Two cups sugar, two and one-half cups water, one-half cup butter, two-thirds cup vinegar, fourteen crackers, one cup raisins, two teaspoons cinnamon, one teaspoon cloves.—*Mrs. P. E. Lacy.*

THANKSGIVING MINCE MEAT.—Five pounds of the round of beef, three pounds of beef suet, six pounds sour apples, four pounds of sugar, two pounds of raisins, two pounds of English currants, four tablespoons ground cinnamon, two tablespoons allspice, two of cloves, four nutmegs, one-half cup salt, one pint molasses, one pint boiled cider. Boil the meat tender and then chop the suet, apples and meat fine, mix them and add a little sweet cider; cook all together. When put between the pastry moisten with sweet cider.—*Miss Alice Daily.*

MINCE PIE.—Three bowls of meat, six bowls of apples, one bowl of molasses, one bowl of vinegar, one bowl of boiled cider, one bowl of suet or butter, two bowls of raisins, five bowls of sugar, one bowl of fruit juice or jelly, two teaspoons each of cinnamon, nutmeg and cloves; one teaspoon each of salt and black pepper. Put together, boil until raisins are tender.—*Mary Bender.*

MOCK MINCE PIES.—Ten round crackers, one cup chopped raisins, one-half cup melted butter, one cup sugar, one cup molasses, one-half cup vinegar (not too strong), two cups hot water, one tablespoon cinnamon, one-half teaspoon cloves, nutmeg.—*Mrs. C. J. Davis.*

PUMPKIN PIE.—One egg, well beaten, one cup brown sugar, one-half cup prepared pumpkin, one-half teaspoon cinnamon, one-fourth teaspoon ginger, butter size of hickory nut, one coffeecup milk. Bake with rich under crust.—*Mrs. Franc E. Gardner.*

PUMPKIN PIE.—Of pumpkin or squash, well stewed, take a large cupful sifted, two eggs, two tablespoons powdered ginger, half teaspoon salt, level cup of sugar, add milk enough to make two pies baked in deep plates. One-quarter cream in the milk is an improvement.—*Mrs. M. W. Howard.*

LEMON PIE.—One lemon, one cup granulated sugar, three eggs, piece of butter size of an egg, two heaping teaspoons of cornstarch. Take the juice of the lemon and one-half cup of water, put on stove to boil. Mix the sugar, butter, cornstarch and yolks of eggs together and stir into the boiling juice. Stir until quite thick. Line pie-tin with rich crust and bake, then fill with the custard. Beat whites of eggs, add two tablespoons of sugar and put on top of pie. Set in the oven to brown.—*Mrs. J. M. Skinner.*

LEMON PIE.—One tablespoon cornstarch, moisten with a very little cold water, add one cup boiling water, one cup sugar, one well-beaten egg, one tablespoon butter, juice and grated rind of one fresh lemon. Bake between two crusts.—*Mrs. Edward Talbort.*

CREAM PIE.—Bake a pie shell of good puff paste. In a double boiler place a cup of sugar and one pint of sweet milk. When boiling stir in two yolks of eggs, and two teaspoons of flour, stir till thick, then beat the whites of two eggs to a stiff froth with a little sugar, spread over top, put in oven and brown. Vanilla flavoring.—*Mrs. E. A. Gilkey.*

MOTHER'S CREAM PIE.—Heat one coffeecup of sweet cream to boiling point in double boiler, then add one tablespoon of flour and one-half cup of sugar moistened with a little cold cream or milk; when thickened set aside to cool. Have pie-plate lined with rich paste and when nearly baked fill with the mixture to which has been added the white of one egg well beaten, a pinch of salt and a little nutmeg. Bake in a moderate oven until custard is set, no longer. Delicious. Much depends on careful baking.—*Mrs. N. B. Jones.*

CREAM PIE.—First, line a pie-tin with crust and bake. Filling for pie: One pint milk, one-half cup sugar, put in a double cooker; when hot add four tablespoons of cornstarch, wet with a little cold milk; let cook fifteen minutes, then add the yolks of two eggs, well beaten, and one tablespoon vanilla; put in crust. Then beat the whites of the eggs to a froth, add three tablespoons sugar; frost pie, brown in oven.—*Mrs. O. E. Spaulding.*

BOSTON CREAM PIE.—Crust, yolks of two eggs and white of one (if whipped cream is used to frost, one egg will do), beaten separately. One-half cup of sugar, one tablespoon of milk or water, three-fourths cup of Royal patent sifted flour, one teaspoon of Queen Flake baking powder; flavor with Jenning's lemon or vanilla. Bake in flat tin in quick oven. When done and cool split with sharp knife.

Cream Filling for Pie.—One-half cup sugar and one-fourth cup Royal patent flour well mixed. One egg well beaten and mixed with flour and sugar. Stir into one-half pint of milk just boiling, add one-half ounce butter and stir until thick. Flavor as above, and spread on crust, frost or cover with whipped cream.—*Mrs. Mary R. Bryant.*

SWEET APPLE PIE.—One cup of grated sweet apple, two eggs, well beaten, a pinch of salt, sweet milk enough to make custard, sweeten and and flavor to suit taste. Bake in one crust. When done add frosting made with the whites of two eggs and two tablespoons of powdered sugar, flavored to suit taste. Set the pie in the oven till frosting is brown.—*Mrs. Alex. Blair.*

CRUMB PIES.—One teacup of bread crumbs, one quart of water, one and one-half cups of sugar, five eggs, two of the whites for frosting, flavor with lemon. This makes three pies.—*Mrs. W. S. Griswold.*

SOUTHERN PIE.—One cup nice raisins, seeded, one cup of granulated sugar, one cup of boiling water, one-half cup of vinegar, one-third of a cup of flour, butter size of small egg, and teaspoon of different spices. —*Marie Henderson.*

Delicious Peach Pie.—Line pie-plate with rich pastry. Mix together flour and sugar, of each one teaspoon, and sprinkle over crust, then fill with peaches peeled and halved. Sprinkle over one-half cup of sugar and one teaspoon flour, with a few bits of butter. Serve with whipped cream.—*Mrs. Franc E. Gardner.*

Pineapple Pie.—Take the weight of one grated pineapple in sugar, and quarter its weight in butter, cream the butter and sugar together, add the well-beaten yolks of five eggs, then a cup of sweet milk and the pineapple, lastly the whites of the eggs beaten to a froth. Bake in one crust only.—*Mrs. P. E. Lacy.*

Rice Pie.—One pint of milk, one-half cup of boiled rice, three spoons of cream, two eggs, four tablespoons of sugar, salt and flavor with Jenning's vanilla.—*Mrs. E. E. Bush.*

Currant Pie.—Take one cup of ripe currants or cherries, mash them, add one cup of sugar, the yolks of two eggs, one tablespoon cornstarch, three of water, mix them and bake with one crust; beat the whites of the eggs, add one tablespoon of sugar, spread over top, brown slightly. Any kind of fruit, or pie-plant, can be used in the same way.—*Charlotte Cook-book.*

Meringue Pie-plant Pie.—One cup of stewed pie-plant, one teaspoon cornstarch or flour, one cupful of sugar, one yolk of egg, one-half teaspoon of butter, small pinch of salt, flavor with Jenning's extract of lemon, mix thoroughly and bake in one crust. Beat the white of the egg to stiff froth with one tablespoon of sugar and spread over the pie when done. Brown lightly in the oven. Equal to lemon pie. Try it. —*Irma T. Jones.*

PUDDINGS.

Dessert of Apples.—Make a rich syrup of a pound of sugar and put into it a pound of finely flavored, ripe sour apples, nicely pared and cored; stew until soft, then mix smoothly with the syrup and pour all into a mould. Stir into a pint of rich cream, or if none, new milk must answer; two well-beaten eggs, half a cup of sugar, and let it just boil up in a farina kettle, then set aside to cool. When cold, take the apples from the mould and pour this cream custard around it and serve. Flavor with vanilla.—*Mrs. C. E. Bement.*

Iced Apples.—Pare and core one dozen large apples; fill with sugar mixed with a little butter and cinnamon or nutmeg, bake until nearly done. Cool, and if possible without breaking, put the apples on another dish, if not possible, pour off the juice. Have some icing prepared, lay it on top and sides and set in the oven a few minutes to brown slightly. Serve with cream.—*Mrs. C. E. Bement.*

Lemon Sponge.—One-half box Cox's gelatine, four eggs, two cups of sugar, juice of three lemons, one pint of boiling water. Cover the gelatine with one-half cup of cold water. Soak for half an hour, then pour over it the boiling water, add the sugar and stir till dissolved, add the lemon juice and strain into tin basin. Put this in cool place to stand until cold and thick, stirring occasionally. Then beat it to a stiff froth with Dover egg beater and add the well-beaten whites of the eggs, beating all until smooth, then turn in mould and set on ice to harden. Serve with whipped cream or vanilla sauce made with one pint of milk, yolks of four eggs, two tablespoons sugar, one teaspoon Jennings' vanilla. Put the milk on to boil in double boiler. Beat the yolks and sugar together until light, then add them to boiling milk. Stir over the fire for two minutes, take off, put in vanilla and set away to cool.—*Mrs. Edward Cahill.*

Genuine English Plum Pudding.—Crumbs of a one-pound loaf of bread, one quart of rich milk scalded and cooled, one pound washed and dried currants, half pound of stoned raisins, three-fourths pound of beef suet, two grated nutmegs, one tablespoon of cinnamon, the grated peel of two oranges or lemons, one-half pound citron, one pound brown sugar. (The brandy and wine prescribed originally may be omitted.) Steamed in a mould or floured bag five or six hours.—*Mrs. M. W. Howard.*

Steam Plum Pudding.—One cup raisins, one cup currants, one cup suet chopped fine, one cup molasses, one cup bread crumbs, one cup hot water, one cup Royal patent flour, one teaspoonful DeLand's soda. Steam three hours. Sauce for same: Cream, one-half cup butter and one-half cup sugar together, flavor, nutmeg or vanilla.—*Mrs. Toolan.*

Plain Plum Pudding.—One cup of suet chopped fine, one cup of molasses, one cup of milk, two cups of raisins, or one of currants and one of raisins, three of Royal patent flour; of soda, cloves and salt one teaspoon of each. Rub the suet well with the flour. Boil two and one-half hours.—*Mrs. Whitehead.*

Fruit Pudding.—One egg, one cup of milk, one-half cup of sugar, one tablespoon butter, two cups flour, two spoons Queen Flake baking powder. Put fruit or jam in cups and fill with the batter and steam. Serve with hard sauce.—*Mrs. R. Dunkin.*

Orange Dessert.—Pare five oranges, cut in thin slices, pour over them a coffeecup of sugar, make a custard of three eggs, one pint of milk, one tablespoon cornstarch and pour over the fruit. Beat the whites of eggs to froth with two tablespoons powdered sugar, pour over custard and brown in the oven. Serve cold.—*Mrs. R. Dunkin.*

Black Pudding.—One cup of molasses, one cup of water, two tablespoons melted butter, one teaspoonful soda, three cups of Royal patent flour, one cup of raisins and currents, mixed spices to taste. Steam three hours.—*Mrs. C. M. Chittenden*

Fruit Pudding.—One egg, one-half cup of sugar, one-fourth cup of butter, one cup of sweet milk, one and two-thirds cups of Royal patent flour, two teaspoons of Queen Flake baking powder, one cup of fruit stirred in last. Steam one-half hour and serve with soft sauce.—*Mrs. Ed. Johns.*

Orange Short-cake.—Mix as for biscuit and bake in a thin round pan, split while hot and butter well, slice the oranges crosswise, removing all seeds and place between the cake and on top, being generous with both oranges and sugar; serve with whipped cream. This is a beautiful, wholesome and delicious dish.

Orange Shortcake.—Beat together one teacup of sugar and one tablespoon of butter; beat three eggs very light and add; sift together two teacups of Royal patent flour and a heaping teaspoon of Queen Flake baking powder with a little salt, add one cup milk, bake in deep tin plates. Peel and slice four oranges and cover with sugar and let stand until ready to put together, split the cakes, put a layer of orange between and sweetened whipped cream on top.—*Mrs. Fred S. Lawrence.*

Brown Pudding.—Two eggs, one-half cup sugar, one-half cup molasses, piece of butter as large as a walnut, one cup of sweet milk, one and a half cups Royal patent flour, two teaspoons Queen Flake baking powder; stir thoroughly and steam for one and a half hours.

Brown Sauce.—One cup of sugar, one tablespoon of butter, two tablespoons of flour, one tablespoon Baker's chocolate, one scant teaspoon of Jenning's vanilla. Stir to a cream, then pour over it two cups of boiling water, stir till smooth.—*Miss Minnie Ross.*

Suet Pudding.—One cup chopped suet, one cup molasses, one cup seeded raisins, one cup milk, sour if you have it; one teaspoon soda, cinnamon and cloves, salt, flour to make a stiff batter, a little stiffer than for cake

Troy Pudding.—One cup suet chopped fine, one and one-half cups raisins, seeded; three and one-half cups flour, one-half cup molasses, one cup milk, one teaspoon soda. Boil three hours.

Sauce.—Five tablespoons sugar, one tablespoon flour, three tablespoons butter, mix and pour over it one cup boiling water, let come to a boil and stir in the juice and grated rind of a lemon.—*Mrs. W. K. Prudden.*

Grandmother's Suet Pudding.—Scald three cups corn meal with one and one-half pints milk. When cool add one cup molasses, one cup chopped suet, a little salt, and if not a thick batter, add milk or meal as occasion requires. Put in a bag, with room to swell, boil three hours in salted water.—*Mrs. Howard.*

Suet Pudding.—One cup of suet, one cup of molasses, one cup of sweet milk, one cup of raisins, three cups of Royal patent flour, one even teaspoon of soda, a little salt. Steam three hours. To be eaten with liquid sauce.

Every Day Sauce.—To one pint of boiling water add one cup sugar, one tablespoon butter, one tablespoon cornstarch, pinch of salt and flavor to taste.

Suet Pudding.—One cup chopped suet, one cup sour milk, one cup molasses, two cups stoned raisins, three cups flour, one teaspoon soda, cinnamon, nutmeg, cloves. Steam three hours.

Sauce.—One heaping teaspoon of cornstarch mixed smooth with water. Pour on this a pint of boiling water and cook thoroughly. Add the well-beaten yolks of two eggs; when cool add the whites beaten to a stiff froth. Flavor with the juice of lemons —*Mrs. George Pratt.*

SUET PUDDING.—One cup molasses, one cup sour milk, four cups flour, one cup raisins, three-quarters pound beef suet chopped fine, two eggs, one teaspoon cinnamon, one teaspoon of cinnamon, one teaspoon soda, a little salt to taste. Steam three hours.

Dip for Pudding.—One-half cup sugar, one tablespoon flour, butter size of an egg. Wet with a little cold water, then pour boiling water over enough to make a thin gravy.—*Mrs. O. E. Spaulding.*

BOILED OR BAKED INDIAN PUDDING.—Ten heaping tablespoons of meal. Moisten with water enough to boil into a thick mush, then thin with three pints of milk, add one-half cup of molasses, three well-beaten eggs, one-half teaspoon of salt, butter size of an egg, one-half teaspoon of cinnamon, tablespoon of ginger. Dissolve a good half teaspoon of soda and stir in. Bake in a moderate oven one and one-half hours, stirring occasionally.—*Mrs. Albert Clark.*

BAKED INDIAN PUDDING.—One quart of milk, three eggs, one and one-half small cups of Indian meal, a lump of butter as large as an egg and a little salt and a cup of molasses. Bake one-half hour.—*Mrs. A. H. Whitehead.*

SUET PUDDING.—One cup of suet chopped fine, sprinkle on a little flour to keep from sticking, two and one-half cups flour, one teaspoon baking powder, one cup chopped apples, one cup raisins, three eggs beaten separately, spice, and add one-half cup molasses, a little salt. Steam and boil two hours; serve with sauce.—*Mrs. Grace C. Greene.*

ANGEL'S HASH.—One-half dozen oranges, one quart of strawberries or red raspberries, one teacup of grated pineapple, add California grapes and slieed bananas. Sweeten to taste and serve with whipped cream.—*Winnie Wessell.*

Fig Pudding.—Six ounces beef suet chopped fine, three-quarters pound grated bread without crust, six ounces sugar, one pound of figs chopped well together, add one cupful sweet milk and nutmeg to taste. Steam three hours. Any kind of sauce that is preferred.—*Mrs. M. W. Howard.*

Puff Pudding.—Three eggs, one pint of milk, half pint of flour, beat the yolks of the eggs, half of the milk and the flour together until light, then add the whites beaten stiff and the other half of milk and flour. Bake in buttered tin. Eat with thin sauce made of butter and sugar thinned with hot water and flavored.—*Mrs. F. B. Lee.*

Graham Pudding.—One cup sour milk, one cup molasses, one and one-half teaspoons soda, one egg, one cup raisins, two cups graham or Flouroigt. Steam two hours. Serve while hot with a hard sauce made as follows: Beat one cup of sugar and one-half cup of the best butter to a white cream, add the white of one egg, beat a little longer, add two teaspoons of Jennings' vanilla, put on ice until wanted.—*Mrs. P. E. Lacy.*

Graham Pudding,—Two cups graham flour, one cup sweet milk, one cup good Porto Rico molasses, one cup of raisins, two teaspoons of soda. Steam for three hours.—*Mrs. J. H. McClure.*

Pudding Sauce.—One tablespoon of Kingsford's cornstarch, one cup of sugar, a pinch of salt, the juice and grated yellow of the rind of one lemon, one egg and butter size of a walnut. Dissolve the cornstarch with cold water, then turn on the starch hot water to thicken. Stir butter, egg, lemon and sugar together, and pour on the mixture the boiling starch.—*Mrs. J. H. McClure.*

Graham Pudding.—Two cups buttermilk, one-half cup molasses, two teaspoons of soda, a pinch of salt. Stir thick as cake with graham flour, add a few raisins or dried fruit. Put in basin and steam two hours. Eat with cream and sugar.—*Mrs. Edward Talbot.*

APPLE FRITTERS —Make a batter with one cup of sweet milk, one teaspoon of sugar, two eggs, whites and yolks beaten separately, two cups of Royal patent flour, one teaspoon of Queen Flake baking powder mixed with the flour. Chop some good tart apples and mix in the batter and fry in hot lard. Serve with maple syrup. These are very nice.—*Mrs. Annie Collins.*

BACHELOR PUDDING.—Pare and remove the cores of two apples (good sized), chop fine, then mix together with one cup cleaned currants and one pint bread crumbs. Beat three eggs and the juice and rind of one lemon, then pour this over the dry ingredients, mix and put into pudding mould. Steam or boil for two hours. Serve hot with a hard or liquid sauce.—*Mrs. Grace C. Greene.*

HONEYCOMB PUDDING.—One-half cup of butter, one-half cup of sweet milk, one-half cup of Royal patent flour, four eggs, one cup of molasses, one teaspoon soda. Put soda in molasses and add to the above. Bake one-half hour and serve with hard sauce.—*Mrs. J. Noaker.*

GRAHAM PUDDING.—Two cups of graham flour, one cup of sweet milk, one cup of molasses, one cup of raisins, two teaspoons of soda, and spices to taste. Steam two hours.—*Mrs. J. Noaker.*

CRUMB PUDDING.—One quart of sweet milk, one pint of bread crumbs, three-fourths cup of sugar, yolks of four eggs, butter size of an egg, grated rind of one lemon. Bake in slow oven. When done, spread over a layer of jelly, whip the whites of eggs to a froth, add one cup of powdered sugar, flavor with the juice of lemons. Pour over the jelly and bake a light brown. Serve cold.

GOOD STEAMED PUDDING.—One cup raisins, one-half cup molasses, one cup warm water, two yolks of eggs, one and one half cups Voigt's Royal patent flour, one teaspoonful soda, steam two hours; use with sauce as follows: One cup sugar, one egg, butter size of a walnut, one tablespoon flour, two tablespoons cold water, stir these into one pint of boiling milk and flavor with Jennings' extract lemon or vanilla.—*Mrs. A. M. Robson.*

APPLE DUMPLINGS.—Put one and one-half cups sugar, two cups water and piece of butter in baking dish, and set on top of stove so it will boil. Take one and one-half cups flour, one teaspoon baking powder, tablespoon lard, mix together with milk so you can roll it out quite thin, cut in pieces and put as much of sliced sour apples as possible in each piece, put edges together and roll in flour, then put them in the hot syrup and bake.—*Mrs. T. E. Potter.*

WASHINGTON PUDDING.—Two cups Royal patent flour, one cup molasses, one cup milk, one teaspoon cinnamon, one of cloves and one teaspoon soda, one-half spoon of salt, two eggs; steam two hours. To be eaten with pudding sauce.—*Mrs. T. E. Potter.*

PEACH PUDDING.—Cover the bottom of a well-buttered baking dish with two layers of peeled peaches, either whole or quartered, pour over them a batter made as follows: One-half cup sugar, three-fourths cup milk, two cups flour, two eggs, butter the size of an egg, one teaspoon of Queen Flake baking powder. Bake three-quarters of an hour or steam one hour.—*Mrs. W. K. Prudden.*

BAKED SWEET APPLE PUDDING.—Pour boiling milk over three cups corn meal, when cool add half-cup molasses, a little salt and two cups of chopped sweet apples. The mass should be a thick batter, to be baked six or more hours in a moderate heat. If a brick oven is available it should stand in over night.—*Mrs. M. W. Howard.*

CREAM PUDDING.—One small spoon of butter, one large spoon of flour, two large spoons of sugar, salt and Jennings' vanilla, the yolks of four eggs. Mix and cook in one pint of milk. When cool stir in the whites of the eggs, when beaten stiff, and bake twenty minutes. Serve immediately with cream and sugar.—*Lılah E. Elder*

KISS PUDDING No. 11.—Yolks of three eggs, half cup of sugar, one and one-half tablespoons cornstarch. Beat this until light. Add to this one pint boiling water and let boil until it thickens, beat the whites of the eggs stiff, add one-half cup sugar and spread over the top and brown.—*Mrs. F. B. Lee*

CUP DUMPLINGS.—One egg, one tablespoon of butter, one cup of sweet milk, one teaspoon of Queen Flake baking powder, Royal patent flour to make a stiff batter. Drop into buttered cups with raspberry jam between. Steam half an hour.

Sauce.—One egg, two tablespoons of boiling milk, one tablespoon of sugar and flavor with nutmeg.—*Mrs. Emma Haskell.*

SNOW PUDDING.—Three tablespoons of cornstarch cooked in one pint of milk. Beat the whites of two eggs, put with the cornstarch, beat well together, put in a mould and set away to cool.

Sauce.—One cup of sweet milk, one tablespoon of sugar, the yolks of two eggs, let this come to a boil. When cold flavor with Jennings' vanilla.—*Mrs. Emma Haskell.*

STEAMED PUDDING.—One cup of sour milk, one cup of molasses, two eggs, one teaspoon soda, one teaspoon of cinnamon, one teaspoon of cloves, a little salt, and Royal patent flour to make a stiff batter. Steam two hours.—*Miss Tillie Bodermer*

QUICK TAPIOCA PUDDING.—Soak one cup of pearl tapioca a few minutes, pour four cups of hot water over it and let it boil until clear, add one cup of sugar, have a cup of apples or peaches prepared, stir in the fruit, set over fire long enough to cook the fruit. Serve while warm with cream and sugar.—*Mrs. P. E. Lacy.*

Pineapple Pudding.—Take slices of sponge cake or bread and a can of pineapple chopped fine, butter a pudding dish and place in the bottom of it slices of cake or bread, then a layer of pineapple, well sprinkled with sugar, and so on till full, having the last cake. Pour over the top a cold custard. Bake slowly two hours. To be eaten with sugar and cream.—*Mrs. John Whiteley.*

Sunday Dessert.—Two oranges pared and cut into small pieces, place in a dish and sprinkle with sugar. One pint of milk, boil and add yolks of two eggs, one tablespoon of cornstarch moistened. Stir constantly and when cooked pour over the oranges. Beat the whites of the eggs, add two tablespoons of sugar and spread over the custard. Brown lightly and serve cold.—*Mrs. C. J. Hazelton, Omaha, Neb.*

Fruit Loaf.—One-half box gelatine, enough cold water to soften gelatine, juice of one lemon, one-half cup of sugar; put lemon, sugar, and gelatine in a bowl, pour over it one cup of hot water. Slice three oranges, the same of bannanas in six cups and fill with the liquid. To be eaten with or without cream.—*Mrs. John Rork.*

Cottage Pudding.—One teacup of sugar, one egg, one teacup of sweet milk, three tablespoons of melted butter, two teaspoons of baking powder. Two and one-half cups of Royal patent flour.

The sauce—One-half cup of sugar and tablespoon of butter; stir to a cream. One and one-half cups boiling water, one large teaspoon cornstarch; add butter and sugar as soon as scalded; white of one egg and juice and rind of one lemon.—*Mrs. Geo. Ritter.*

Mrs. Storr's Pudding Sauce.—Two eggs beaten separately, one teacup of powdered sugar, four tablespoons of milk, one teaspoon of Jennings' vanilla. After beating the eggs put the yolks and whites together, add the sugar and vanilla, and beat thoroughly. Just before serving add the milk. This is not to be cooked but serve cold.

SOUR SAUCE FOR PUDDINGS.—Four tablespoons of sugar, one of butter, one of flour, one-half cup of boiling water, boil one minute and add vinegar to suit.—*Winnie Wessell.*

FRUIT CREAM.—One-third of a box of gelatine dissolved in one-fourth pint of water, three-fourths pint fruit juice, whites of three eggs, one-half pint of whipped cream, sugar according to kind of fruit, if juice is too sweet add lemon juice. Place juice and sugar together and warm slightly, add dissolved gelatine (strained), set in a cold place until it begins to jelly, whip gelatine and juice until light, before adding eggs and cream. Then add the whites of the eggs beaten with a little pulverized sugar and last of all, the whipped cream. Pile in a fruit dish or place in moulds. If pineapple is used the fruit chopped fine and added last is very nice.—*Mrs. C. J. Davis.*

PINEAPPLE FLOAT.—One pint of water, juice and pulp of two lemons, one coffeecup of sugar, when boiling add four tablespoons of cornstarch dissolved in cold water, let it boil fifteen minutes, stirring constantly. When cool pour over pineapple picked fine with a fork. On the top spread beaten whites of three eggs. Sweeten and flavor as you like.—*Mrs. F. B. Lee.*

Use Knox's Sparkling Gelatine.

PINEAPPLE CREAM.—One pint of cream whipped stiff, one cup of sugar. Soak one-half box of gelatine in one cup of milk until thoroughly dissolved, one fresh pineapple (or one can of pineapple), added to the cream, when gelatine is cool add the cream, sugar and apple, pour into a mould and set away to stiffen. Cocoanut may be used in place of pineapple, using half cup of cocoanut.—*Mrs. Ellen Westcott.*

HAMBURG CREAM.—Take grated rind and juice of two large lemons, the same of oranges, one-half teacup of water, two teacups of sugar, a piece of butter, tablespoonful, one tablespoon of cornstarch dissolved and strained into the above until thoroughly cooked over steam, then add the yolks of five eggs well beaten, let cool a little and stir in lightly the whites of five eggs whipped to stiff froth, dish into cups or glasses to cool.—*Mrs. Earl.*

Bavarian Cream.—One-half box gelatine soaked in one-half cup of cold water one hour, crush one quart any kind of berries and put through a sieve to remove seeds, add to the berries one cup of sugar, put gelatine in a bowl over a kettle of boiling water; when dissolved add the berry juice, stir and place in a basin on ice, or where it will cool. Add one pint of whipped cream. When thoroughly mixed pour into a mould and set away to harden.

For raspberry cream use one pint of raspberry juice, one-half cup of sugar and follow the above rules.—*Mrs. Ellen Westcott.*

Spanish Cream.—One-half box of gelatine dissolved in one-half pint of milk, take the remainder of one quart of milk, let it come to boiling, stir in the gelatine, two eggs (yolks only) well beaten, one cup sugar, salt, one lemon (juice only), whites of two eggs beaten to a stiff froth, flavor to taste. The lemon juice and whites of eggs to be beaten in the last thing before pouring into the moulds. The heat must be kept up till all the ingredients are added excepting the whites of egg and lemon juice.—*Mrs. H. B. Baker.*

Orange Pudding.—Juice of jour oranges, add equal amount of water, one cup of sugar, boil and thicken with two tablespoons cornstarch. Mould and serve with whipped cream.—*Mrs. Chas. W. Gilkey.*

Orange Pudding.—One quart of milk, three eggs, two dessertspoonfuls of cornstarch; use the yolks, cornstarch and milk, and make a boiled custard; let it stand until cold. Pare and slice four oranges in a dish with one cup of sugar, pour the custard over the oranges, stir all together, then put the whites, well beaten with a little sugar on the top of the whole, set in oven for a few moments to brown. Let it get very cold before serving.—*Mrs. C. J. Davis.*

Rice Balls.—Take boiled rice, mould it in cups, make a custard of one quart of milk, four well-beaten eggs, one cup sugar, cook until it thickens; when cool add flavoring, pour over the rice.—*Mrs. E. E. Bush.*

Rice Pudding.—Put one cup rice, one teaspoon salt, one quart milk in a covered pail, let it boil in water one and three-fourths hours, then stir in the yolks of four eggs, and one cup sugar; beat the whites to a froth, flavor and put on the pudding; place in the oven and let it remain long enough to brown.—*Mrs. E. H. Whitney.*

Sue's Way to Cook Rice.—Wash one cup of rice and dry it; three pints water and a little salt, let come to a boil, then add the rice and boil twelve minutes, keep covered, drain off the water and set on the back of the stove ten minutes, with the cover partly off; then cover a few moments.—*Mrs. C. M. Chittenden.*

Rice Pudding Without Eggs —Two quarts of milk, one-half teacup of rice, one cup of sugar, half cup of raisins, wash the rice and put it with the rest of the ingredients into the milk, bake slowly from two to three hours (spoiled if over-baked); stir two or three times the first hour of baking. If properly done this pudding is delicious. To be eaten cold.—*Mrs. F. B. Lee.*

Lemon Rice.—Boil one-half pint of rice in one quart of milk until very soft, add to it while hot the yolks of three eggs, grated rind of one lemon, five tablespoonfuls of sugar, a pinch of salt, if too thick add more milk; pour into a pudding dish, beat whites of the eggs very stiff, add eight tablespoonfuls of pulverized sugar, the juice of two lemons, brown lightly on top. Serve cold.—*Marie M. Henderson.*

ORANGE CHARLOTTE.—One-third box of gelatine in one-third cup cold water, add one-third cup boiling water, one cup sugar, juice of one lemon, one cup orange juice and pulp, whites of three eggs; line bowl with sections of orange; when the gelatine with sugar, orange and water begins to stiffen, beat in the beaten whites and mould. Serve with whipped cream.—*Miss Martha Buck.*

AMBROSIA.—One grated cocoanut, ten oranges picked to shreds, one pound of powdered sugar. Very nice to serve with ice cream.—*Mrs. Marvin.*

Use Knox's Sparkling Gelatine.

SNOW PUDDING.—One-half box gelatine dissolved in one pint of boiling water. When nearly cool add one cup of sugar, juice of one lemon, and strain; add whites of three eggs beaten well, then beat all together very thoroughly. Pour into moulds and serve with custard made with yolks of three eggs, half a teaspoon of cornstarch, one-half cup of sugar and one pint of boiling milk.—*Marie M. Henderson.*

PRUNE PUDDING.—One pound stewed prunes, whites of four eggs, one cup sugar. After prunes are stewed drain off juice, remove the stones and chop. Beat eggs very stiff, add the sugar gradually, beating all the time, then stir in chopped prunes. Bake twenty minutes and serve cold with whipped cream or cream and sugar.—*Mrs. J. E. Nichols.*

FIG DESSERT.—Boil a quantity of figs in a little water until they can be pierced with a straw. Set aside to cool. Serve very cold with whipped cream.—*Mrs. Neenah Keavy, Detroit.*

PRUNE WHIP.—Soak one-half pound of prunes over night. In the morning stew them slowly till very soft. Sweeten while stewing, then mash them to a paste, after removing the stones. Take the whites of six eggs, sweeten a little to take off the raw taste of the egg, then beat thoroughly the eggs and prunes, mixing as lightly as possible. Bake one-half hour in a slow oven until a delicate brown. Serve with whipped cream or thin custard.—*Mrs. W. C. Edwards, Dowagiac.*

PRUNE WHIP.—Soak twenty prunes over night and stew in the morning in as little water as possible. Remove stones and chop. Beat the whites of four eggs and stir in the prunes with two tablespoons of sugar. Bake twenty minutes, serve with whipped cream or frosted.—*Mrs. J. M. Earle.*

Use Knox's Sparkling Gelatine.

APPLE PUFF.—One cup of baked apple, one cup of sugar and whites of two eggs beaten thoroughly together. Use the yolks of the two eggs and one-half the sugar with one pint of milk for custard and pour over the apple. Very nice.—*Mrs. Mary J. Earle.*

PEACH BAVARIAN CREAM.—Cover one-half box gelatine with one-half pint of cold water and soak one-half hour. Press one pint of canned peaches through a sieve or colander and sweeten well. Stir the gelatine over boiling water until dissolved. Whip a pint of cream stiff, add gelatine and peaches and turn into a clean basin which you must stand on cracked ice while you stir until it stiffens. Then add the whipped cream, mix thoroughly, turn into a mould to cool and serve with whipped cream piled around the base after you have turned the contents of the mould into a pretty dish.

CHARLOTTE RUSSE.—One pound lady fingers, one quart sweet cream, three-fourths cup powdered sugar, two teaspoons vanilla. Split fingers and fit neatly in bottom and sides of moulds. Whip cream to stiff froth, sweeten and flavor and fill moulds. Lay fingers closely together on top. Set on ice till used. You may use sponge cake, cutting it in thin strips for sides, leaving crust for bottom and top in place of lady fingers —*Mrs. F. G. Clark.*

CHARLOTTE RUSSE.—Beat one pint of cream till thick and foamy; beat the whites of four eggs to a stiff froth. Soak two tablespoons of Knox's gelatine in two tablespoons of cold water one hour, then add two of boiling water; let it cool, add to the cream two-thirds cup of pulverized sugar, flavor with vanilla, stir in the eggs, last the gelatine; beat with egg beater until well blended. Pour into moulds lined with lady fingers. In summer double the quantity of gelatine must be used.—*Mrs. E. Marvin.*

Use Knox's Sparkling Gelatine.

CHERRY BLANC MANGE.—Take one quart of canned cherries, one-half box Knox's Sparkling gelatine dissolved in one-half glass of water; heat the cherries and gelatine together, sugar to taste, flavor with a few drops lemon juice. Pour into a mould which has been rinsed in cold water. Serve cold with whipped cream.

COFFEE MANGE.—One cup of very strong coffee, one cup of sugar, one cup of cream, one-half box Knox's Sparkling gelatine dissolved in two cups of milk over the fire, add cream last, after the rest is cold. Serve with whipped cream.—*Miss Edith Collins, Charlotte.*

CHARLOTTE RUSSE.—Soak one-fourth box of gelatine in one-half cup milk one hour; when dissolved set cup in hot water using gelatine luke warm, into one pint whipped cream add one-half cup pulverized sugar, a little salt and the beaten whites of two eggs and flavor with vanilla, then add gelatine and strain while pouring in. Stir until gelatine is well mixed with cream and when nearly stiff enough to drop, turn into mould lined with lady fingers or narrow slices of sponge cake having cake even at top, first dipping cake in white of egg. Use Knox's Sparkling gelatine.

APPLE RUSSE.—Fill a pudding dish with quartered apples, cover with bits of butter, one cup of sugar and a little cinnamon. Bake brown and serve with whipped cream.—*Saginaw Cook Book.*

PEACH PUDDING.—One pint stale bread, one quart milk, one-fourth cup butter, one-half cup sugar, one saltspoon salt, four eggs, six or eight peaches. Grate the inside of a loaf, and soak it in the hot milk. Pare, halve and stone the peaches, and place them, the hollow side up, in a buttered mould. Cream the butter, add the sugar, salt, eggs well beaten, and stir all into the milk. Pour it over the peaches, cover, and place the mould in a pan of hot water in the oven and bake two hours. Serve with creamy sauce.—*Am. Kitchen Magazine.*

Use Knox's Sparkling Gelatine.

PEACH TAPIOCA.—One-half cup pearl tapioca, one saltspoon salt, one pint boiling water, one-fourth cup sugar, ripe peaches. Cook in a double boiler till the tapioca is dissolved. Add the sugar and one cup of peaches sliced and mashed. Pare six peaches, cut them in halves, remove the stone and place them, the cleft side up, in a dish for serving. Pour the tapioca over them, and serve very cold with sugar and cream. —*Am. Kitchen Magazine.*

PEACH CREAM.—Take a can of peaches and cut the fruit into small pieces. Dissolve one-fourth box of gelatine in hot water, having first soaked it in cold water. Whip one-half pint cream until it is solid, add the gelatine, and sugar to taste; stir in the peaches and pour into moulds to form. A very little salt put in the cream before whipping is an improvement. Use Knox's Sparkling gelatine.

ANGEL FOOD PUDDING.—Whites of six eggs well beaten, pulverized sugar, tablespoonful to an egg beat in, six tablespoons of currant jelly beat in. Put on ice and serve with whipped cream.—*Miss Martha Buck.*

GLAIZED APPLES WITH CREAM.—For a dozen large apples use one and one-half cups of water. Put one cup of sugar in a saucepan with the water and boil rapidly for twenty minutes. Pare and core the apples, keeping them whole; put them in deep earthen plates and put a teaspoon of sugar in the center of each apple, baste the outside of each apple with one-half teaspoon of hot syrup, place the pans in a moderately hot oven and bake the fruit until it is tender, basting frequently with the syrup. When the apples are done place them on a flat dish and pour over them the juice from the pan in which they were baked. Serve cold, with bowl of whipped cream.

LEMON CUSTARD.—One lemon grated, rind and juice; yolks of four eggs, four tablespoons of sugar, two of water. Let it simmer a little, then add the whites and two tablespoons of sugar.—*Mrs. Whitney.*

RICE CREAM.—Beat into one pint of whipped cream one cup boiled rice, not quite cold, and a large tablespoon of gelatine, dissolved. Put in a mould and serve with sauce. Use Knox's Sparkling gelatine.

Sauce.—Make a rich white sugar syrup and add a glass of orange marmalade.

FROZEN PUDDING (twenty dishes).—Swell two tablespoons of gelatine in a little water, two eggs beaten, stir in one and one-half cups of granulated sugar, sift in one tablespoon flour, heat one pint milk (over water) hot and stir in the egg, sugar and gelatine till it boils. Remove from stove, turn in one quart of cream and as it freezes stir in crystallized fruit and one pound of hot sliced citron. Use Knox's Sparkling gelatine.—*Lilah E. Elder.*

RAISIN PUFFS.—Two eggs, one cup of sugar, one-half cup of butter, one cup of sweet milk, one cup of raisins, two cups of flower, three teaspoons of Queen Flake baking powder. Put in cups and steam half an hour. Serve with soft sauce.—*Mrs. Geo. Ritter.*

APPLE CREAM.—Pare, quarter, core and boil six large tart apples in a pint of water, press through a sieve, add one cup of sugar, two teaspoons Jennings' vanilla, the beaten whites of three eggs; beat hard while one-half package Knox's Sparkling gelatine is dissolving in one pint of water, mix well together and pour into moulds. Serve with whipped cream.

Apple Dip.—Take three large tart apples, pare and slice very fine in your baking dish, add a small piece of butter and two tablespoons sugar, Then take one egg, two tablespoons sugar, one-half cup sweet milk, two tablespoons butter, one cup flour, one teaspoon baking powder. Beat this together and pour over apples and bake.—*Mrs. C. C. Wood.*

Coffee Jelly.—Soak one box of gelatine two hours in one-half pint of cold water, then pour on it one and one-half pints of boiling water. When wholly dissolved add one pint of sugar and one pint strong coffee. Strain the jelly and pour into a mould to harden. When served, put into a dish with whipped cream around it. The cream should be sweetened a very little. Use Knox's Sparkling gelatine.

Lemon Jelly.—One package Knox's Sparkling gelatine, one cup lemon juice or four lemons, two and one-half cups of sugar, two quarts of water. Dissolve the gelatine in one pint of water, add the other three pints of boiling water, the lemon juice and sugar. Strain into moulds and set in a cool place to harden.—*Mrs. C. J. Davis.*

Nut Ambrosia.—To half box Knox's Sparkling gelatine add one quart hot water. Let this stand until thoroughly dissolved, then add juice of four lemons. Let all come to a good boil; when just cool, add one pound blanched almonds chopped fine, then on top lay one-half pound candied cherries and serve with whipped cream.

ICES.

Apricot Ice.—To the juice of two lemons allow eight apricots or even ten, if small. Remove the skins, blanch and pound to a paste a few of the kernels, then add one-half pint water and two ounces fine sugar. Let this stand in an earthen jar or punch-bowl for an hour and a half, then strain. After it is strained, stir in the whites of three eggs beaten to a stiff froth with four ounces of powdered sugar, and then freeze. To serve with rich cake nothing is nicer for an "afternoon" or luncheon. Canned apricots will do.

Lemon Ice.—The juice of four lemons, three pints of thin syrup made with less than a pint of sugar. When cold add the lemon juice, and when partly frozen stir in the whites of two eggs beaten very light with a little powdered sugar, scarcely a small tablespoonful.—*Mrs. Marvin.*

Orange Ice.—One quart of water, one quart sugar boiled together and let stand until cold; dissolve two tablespoons of Knox's Sparkling gelatine in a teacup of warm water, add the juice of six oranges and three lemons and strain; just before putting into the freezer, add the whites of two eggs beaten stiff.

Lemon Sherbet.—The juice of five lemons, one pint of sugar, one quart water, one tablespoon gelatine. Soak the gelatine in a little of the water, boil one cup of the water and dissolve the gelatine in it. Mix together the sugar, water, gelatine and lemon juice, turn into the can and freeze. This is light and creamy.—*Mrs. J. E. St. John.*

Use Knox's Sparkling Gelatine.

Ice Cream.—One quart of cream, one pint of milk, one pint of powdered sugar, one tablespoon of Jennings' vanilla and whites of four eggs.

Raspberry Vinegar.—Put the red raspberries in a porcelain kettle, cover with highland vinegar to extract the juice, let them heat, mashing with a spoon; then cool before pressing the juice through a coarse cloth. To each quart of juice add one pint of vinegar. Put this mixture in the preserving kettle with one pound (scant) sugar to each pint. Boil ten minutes, taking off all the scum that may rise, and bottle. It will keep for years if well sealed. About two tablespoonfuls in a glass of icewater makes a refreshing drink.—*Saginaw "Sweets to the Sweet."*

Fruit Ice.—One-half can apricots, three bananas, three oranges, three cups of sugar, three lemons, three cups of water. Put a sieve over a large bowl, turn in the apricots, and rub all but the skin through. Peel the bananas, remove seeds and dark portions and sift the pulp,

pour the water in gradually to help the pulp go through the strainer. Squeeze the oranges and lemons and strain through into the fruit pulp. Add sugar and when dissolved freeze.—*Mrs. J. Sibbald, Saginaw.*

CURRANT SHERBET.—One pint sugar, one quart of water, one pint of currant juice, the juice of one lemon. Boil the water and sugar together half an hour; add the current and lemon juice to the syrup; let this cool and freeze.

PINEAPPLE ICE.—For one-gallon freezer take one quart granulated sugar, one quart water, boil to thick syrup and pour boiling hot over one can grated pineapple, add the juice and pulp of four lemons and put into freezer (I think it nicer strained), add the stiffly-beaten whites of three eggs, fill up with water, lacking one quart; put to freeze while hot.—*Viola G. Moffett.*

Use Knox's Sparkling Gelatine.

CAKE.

"Cooking is a fine art, to which you must bring common sense and judgment."

WEDDING CAKE.—Ten eggs, whites and yolks beaten separately; two pounds of stoned raisins, two pounds currants, one pound sugar, one pound flour, one cup of milk, half pound citron shredded fine; salt, cloves, cinnamon, allspice, used with judgment; two teaspoons Queen Flake baking powder. Bake in two loaves about four hours in a moderately heated oven.—*Mrs. M. W. Howard.*

TIN WEDDING CAKE.—Rub one cup butter and three cups of sugar to a cream, add one cup of milk and four of flour, five eggs, two teaspoons of baking powder, quarter pound of citron. This makes two loaves.—*Mrs. C. M. Chittenden.*

"MAUD S." CAKE.—Make a custard of eight tablespoons grated chocolate, five tablespoons sugar, one-half cup of sweet milk, boil until thick. While custard is cooking stir one-half cup butter, one and one-half cups of brown sugar, three eggs, drop in one at a time and beat each well, and one-half cup of Royal patent flour; stir in custard; add one and one-half cups flour with two teaspoons of Queen Flake baking powder, one-fourth cup of sweet milk; flavor with Jennings' vanilla; bake in layers. Use boiled frosting with a little chocolate grated in. Filling: One cup sugar, three tablespoons of water, white of one egg well beaten, cool sugar enough not to cook egg, beat well, grate in little chocolate.—*Mrs. William Donovan.*

SNOW CAKE.—Two-cups pulverized sugar and one cup butter beaten to a cream, one cup sweet milk, three cups of flour, two teaspoons baking powder, whites of eight eggs. Flavor to taste.—*Mrs. R. B. Kellogg.*

FEATHER CAKE.—Two scant cups sifted flour, two tablepoons of Queen Flake baking powder, one tablespoon of butter, one cup of sugar, one cup of milk, one egg, one to two teaspoons Jennings' vanilla. Sift flour and baking powder together. Cream butter, beat in sugar and add flavoring, then the milk, and egg, beaten to a foam. Stir in the flour quickly and bake in a shallow pan in a quick oven. Bake in layers.—*Mrs. M. W. Bement.*

CHOCOLATE MARBLE CAKE.—Whites of two eggs, one cup of granulated sugar, one tablespoon of butter, one-half cup of milk, two cups of Royal patent flour, two teaspoons of baking powder, one scant teaspoon of vanilla. Cream sugar and butter by adding a little sugar at a time. After all is well mixed, beat hard five minutes, then take half of the batter out into another dish, add two tablespoons of grated Baker's chocolate, stir well and place alternate layers of white and dark in the baking tin.—*Miss Minnie Ross.*

MAPLE SUGAR CAKE.—One cup butter, two of sugar, three of Voigt's

Royal patent flour, four eggs, one cup milk. Bake in layers, and use the following filling between two and over the top: Take one cup maple sugar, melt and boil until it hairs, beat the white of one egg to a stiff froth, add the sugar, a little at a time, and beat until cold.—*Mrs. Edward Talbort.*

EGGLESS CAKE.—Two cups buttermilk, two cups sugar, two cups chopped raisins, one cup butter, four cups Royal patent flour, cinnamon, nutmeg, cloves and soda, each one tablespoonful. This makes two cakes. —*Mrs. Talbort.*

Use Knox's Sparkling Gelatine.

SPICE CAKE.—One and one-half cups of sugar, three-fourths cup of butter, four eggs (keep whites of two for frosting), one cup of sweet milk, two cups of Royal patent flour, two teaspoons of Queen Flake baking powder, one teaspoon of cinnamon, one teaspoon of cloves, one-half teaspoon of allspice. Bake in dripping pan. For frosting, boil two cups of sugar till it hairs, and then pour over the whites of the two eggs that have been beaten a very little. Beat this until it is very smooth and nearly cold.—*Ella W. Shank.*

SURPRISE CAKE.—One egg, one cup of sugar, one-half cup of butter, sweet milk one cup, soda one teaspoon, cream of tartar two teaspoons. Flavor with Jennings' lemon extract and use sufficient sifted Royal patent flour to make the proper consistency, not too stiff.

"ANGEL'S FOOD."—The "knack" in making angel's food is to beat the eggs (with wire spoon) long and hard till they "stand alone," then add vanilla, and having sifted flour, sugar, cream of tartar and a pinch of salt the required number of times together, add all at once, stirring very little, just enough to mix and hardly that. A pan with tube is much best, and the oven must be very "moderate."—*Julia B. Judson.*

ANGEL CAKE.—Whites of nine large fresh eggs or ten small one, one and one-fourth cups sifted granulated sugar, one cup sifted flour, a pinch of salt, one-half teaspoon cream tartar. After sifting flour four or five times, measure and set aside one cup, then sift and measure one and one-fourth cups granulated sugar, beat egg about half, add cream of tartar and beat very stiff, then flour lightly and flavor to taste. Put in pan and in oven at once. Moderate heat. Will bake in thirty-five to fifty minutes.—***Mrs. W. H. Porter.***

GOLD LAYER.—Large one-half cup butter, large one-half cup sweet skimmed milk, one heaping cup of granulated sugar (all you can crowd on) two and one-half cups flour, six yolks, two heaping teaspoons baking powder, stir very lightly. Hot oven. This is nice to use up the eggs.—***Mrs. W. H. Porter.***

Use Knox's Sparkling Gelatine.

WASHINGTON CAKE.—One and one-half cups sugar, one-half cup butter, one cup milk, two and two-thirds cups of flour, whites of three eggs, two teaspoons Queen Flake baking powder. Very nice baked in a loaf cake or for any kind of layer cake.—***Mrs. M. E. Marvin.***

A SIMPLE FIG CAKE.—Two cups of sugar, one-half cup of butter, one-half cup of sweet milk, four eggs, whites only, beaten to a froth; two cups flour, two teaspoons baking powder, one-half pound figs chopped. Make a syrup with little water, figs and sugar, cook and put between layers.—***Mrs. W. Donovan.***

COFFEE CAKE.—One cup of sugar, one-half cup of molasses, one cup of butter, one cup of cold coffee, one and one-half cups raisins, one teaspoon soda, one teaspoon cloves, two teaspoons cinnamon, four cups of flour.—***Mrs. H. P. Bartlett.***

PORK CAKE.—One pound of fat pork chopped very fine, one pint boiling water, put on while boiling hot; when cold add a teaspoon of soda, seven cups of flour, two cups sugar, one cup molasses, two pounds of raisins and other fruit if wanted, spice to taste.

BREAD CAKE.—Two and one-half cups of light dough, one and one-half cups of granulated sugar, one cup of butter, one teaspoon of soda, one cup of raisins, three eggs, one-half teaspoon of cinnamon. Bake in a slow oven.

CORNSTARCH CAKE.—One cup of sugar, one-half cup butter, scant, beat to a cream; beat the whites of three eggs and add to the butter and sugar, add one-half cup of cornstarch with one-half teaspoon Queen Flake baking powder in it, one-half cup sweet milk, one and one-half cups of Royal patent flour sifted with one teaspoon baking powder.—*Mrs. R. K. Bryan.*

WHITE CAKE.—Two-thirds of a cup of butter, one and one-half cups of sugar, two-thirds cup of sweet milk, three cups of flour, one teaspoonful of lemon extract, two teaspoonfuls of baking powder, whites of seven eggs.—*Mrs. W. W. Armstrong.*

WHITE CAKE.—One and one-half cups of sugar, one-half cup of butter, one half cup of sweet milk, two teaspoons of Cream Flake baking powder, two and one-half cups of Voigt's Royal patent flour, season with Jennings' lemon or vanilla, add last the whites of four eggs whipped to a stiff froth. Stir thoroughly and bake in a moderate oven.—*Mrs. J. H. McClure.*

Use Knox's Sparkling Gelatine.

WHITE CAKE—One cup confectioner's sugar, one-third cup butter, one-half cup milk, two scant cups Voigt's Royal patent flour, two teaspoons Queen Flake baking powder, whites of three eggs last; flavoring. —*Bessie Marble.*

PATTY CAKES.—(Excellent.)—Cream, one-half cup butter, slowly add one cup sugar, one-half cup sweet milk, the beaten yolks of two eggs, then the beaten whites of two eggs. Sift in one heaping cup flour, one teaspoon baking powder, one heaping tablespoon cinnamon.

CREAM PUFFS.—One cup water, one-half cup of butter; when boiling stir in one cup sifted Royal patent flour; when cold add three eggs, well beaten, then beat the whole and drop in tins and bake for twenty-five minutes.

Custard for Puffs.—One cup sweet milk, one egg, one tablespoon cornstarch, one cup sugar, Jennings' vanilla.—*Mrs. P. E. Lacy.*

FRUIT CAKE —One cup of brown sugar and one of molasses, one-half cup of butter, one-half cup of sour milk two and one-half cups of Royal patent flour, yolks of four eggs, one-half teaspoon of each of cloves, allspice cinnamon and nutmeg. One teaspoon of soda added to the sour milk, then stir in one pound of raisins and one of currants, one-quarter pound of citron, all well dredged with one teacup of flour. Bake in a slow oven till well done.—*Mrs. C. P. Lesher.*

PLAIN FRUIT CAKE.—Five eggs, three cups dark brown sugar, one cup sour milk, one teaspoon soda, one cup New Orleans molasses, one-half teaspoon allspice, one and one-half teaspoons of cloves, four cups of Royal patent flour; add, dredged with the flour, one and one-half pounds of raisins and some currants.—*Miss Elizabeth O'Connor.*

FARMER'S FRUIT CAKE.—Soak three cups of dried apples over night in warm water. Chop (slightly) in the morning, then simmer two hours in two cups molasses, add two eggs, one cup sugar, one cup sweet milk, three-fourths cup butter, one and one-half teaspoons soda, Voigt's Royal patent flour to make thick batter, spice to suit the taste. Bake in quick oven.—*Mrs. C. J. Davis.*

SPICE FRUIT CAKE.—Two cups brown sugar, one cup butter, one cup sour milk, three cups flour, one cup raisins (chop fine), two eggs, one teaspoon of soda, season with cloves and cinnamon.—*Mrs. Dr. J. Lamoreaux.*

WHITE FRUIT CAKE.—One cup of butter, two cups of sugar, two and one-half cups of flour, two-thirds of cup of sweet milk, whites of six eggs, one pound of blanched almonds, chopped, one pound citron, sliced thin, one pound of seedless raisins, one and one-half teaspoonfuls of Queen Flake baking powder. It will take two pounds of almonds before shelling.—*Mrs. W. W. Armstrong.*

LAYER CAKES.

Marsh Mallow Cake.—Two cups sugar, one-half cup butter, one cup milk, two and one-half cups Royal patent flour, whites of four eggs, two teaspoons Queen Flake baking powder, one-fourth teaspoon rose water.

Frosting: Two cups powdered sugar, one-half cup water. Boil together until it strings from spoon, have ready whites of two eggs beaten, one-half pound marsh mallows. Split in half, spread between layers on top of frosting while cake is hot.—*Mrs. Jessie M. Turner.*

Spiced Layer Cake.—Two cups brown sugar, two-thirds cup butter, one cup sweet milk, two and one-fourth cups Royal patent flour, yolks of five eggs, three teaspoons baking powder, one teaspoon cinnamon, one teaspoon cloves, one teaspoon nutmeg, one teaspoon allspice, one cup chopped raisins in frosting, vanilla in both cake and frosting.—*Carrie Jones.*

Spice Layer Cake.—One cup brown sugar, one-half cup of butter, one-half cup of sour milk, two cups of flour, three eggs, save out white of one for frosting, one teaspoon of soda, one teaspoon of spice to taste, one teaspoon of Queen Flake baking poder.—*Mrs. Chas. W. Gilkey.*

Chocolate Layer Cake.—One cup of sugar, one-half cup butter, two eggs, one-half cup of sweet milk, two cups of Voigt's Royal patent flour, two spoonfuls Queen Flake baking powder.

Filling: One-half cake of chocolate grated and dissolved in a small cup of milk, let boil, then add one-half cup of sugar, a small piece of butter, a pinch of salt and Jennings' vanilla flavoring.—*Mrs. Annis Collins.*

French Cream Cake.—One cup sugar, three eggs, two tablespoons cold water, one teaspoon Queen Flake baking powder, one and one-half cups Royal patent flour. Bake in quick oven.

Filling.—Scald one pint of milk, dissolve two tablespoons of cornstarch in a little milk, beat this with two eggs and one cup sugar, stir into the boiling milk and when it boils add one tablespoon butter and Jennings' vanilla, stir until quite smooth, split the cake while hot and spread with the cream.—*Mrs. E. E. Bush.*

Brown Raisin Layer Cake.—Half cup of sugar, half cup molasses, half cup of sour milk, half cup butter, two eggs, one-half teaspoon of soda, a little salt, nutmeg and cinnamon, Royal patent flour to mix a stiff batter. Chop one-half cup of seeded raisins and mix with frosting for filling. *Mrs. W. S. Wright.*

Molasses Layer Cake.—Three cups Royal patent flour, two teaspoonfuls Queen Flake baking powder, one saltspoonful salt, one tablespoonful butter, one-half cup molasses, two yolks of eggs, one-half cup sugar, one teaspoonful each ginger and cinnamon, one cup milk. Sift together flour, salt and baking powder. Cream butter and sugar, add yolks of eggs, molasses and spices, then milk and prepared flour. Bake in three layers.

Filling.—Whites two eggs, two cups confectioner's sugar and dessertspoonful hot water, stir thoroughly and flavor with a teaspoon of Jennings' lemon or vanilla. When smooth, spread between layers; cover top with same.—*Mrs. M. W. Bement.*

Caramel Filling for Cake.—One cup sugar, one cup thick sour cream. Boil together until as thick as frosting; beat until cold.—*Mrs. Chas. Broas.*

Coffee Filling for Cake.—To one-half cup of strong coffee add two cups of white sugar; boil five minutes, set in a pan of cold water and stir until creamy. Spread on quickly; the cake must be cold before frosting is put on.—*Mrs. H. R. Pratt.*

Chocolate Frosting.—One square of melted chocolate, whites of two eggs well beaten, nine tablespoons of pulverized sugar.—*Winnie Wessell.*

Chocolate Frosting.—One cup granulated sugar, one-half cup of cream, one square of chocolate (grated), cook until thick, cool and add Jennings' vanilla, spread on cake.—*Mrs. C. J. Davis.*

Chocolate Frosting.—One cup sugar, five tablespoons of milk, boil five minutes, always boil one minute for every tablespoon of milk, then add from one-half to a whole square of bitter chocolate, then stir till cold. It will be fine-grained and creamy.—*Miss Lizzie O'Connor.*

COOKIES AND MOLASSES CAKE.

HERMITS.—Two cups of light brown sugar, one cup of butter, three eggs, one-half teaspoon of soda, three tablespoons sour milk, one cup chopped raisins, one teaspoon of cinnamon, one-half teaspoon cloves, same of nutmeg. Roll thin and cut with cooky cutter. These will keep for months.—*Mrs. G. L. Freeman*

HERMITS.—One and one-half cups of brown sugar, two eggs, one-half cup of butter. two teaspoons of sour milk, one level teaspoon of different spices, one cupful of currants.—*Mrs. Ed. Johns.*

FRUIT COOKIES.—One and one-half cups sugar, one cup of butter, three eggs, one-half cup of sour milk, one small teaspoon of soda, one teaspoon cinnamon, one half teaspoon of cloves, a little nutmeg, one cup of chopped raisins, can use part currants or dried cherries, stir stiff and drop on buttered tins.—*Mrs. C. A. Gower.*

FRUIT COOKIES.—Two cups sugar, one cup sour milk, one cup butter, one cup English currants, two eggs, one teaspoon of soda, one-half nutmeg and add flour. Mix soft; bake quick.—*Mrs. George Spaulding.*

CHOCOLATE WAFERS.—One cup brown sugar, one of white sugar, one of butter, two eggs, one cup of grated chocolate, one teaspoon of Jennings' vanilla, enough Royal patent flour to make quite stiff (about two cups), roll very thin, cut in squares and bake quickly.—*Mrs. E. E. Bush.*

WHITE COOKIES.—Heaping cup of sugar, two eggs, one cup of butter, one-half cup of sweet milk, two teaspoons of baking powder. Bake quick, and not mix too stiff.—*Mame Dillon.*

WHITE COOKIES.—Two cups sugar, one cup of butter, three eggs, scant half cup sour milk, half teaspoon soda, one nutmeg. Do not mix too stiff.—*Mrs. R. B. Kellogg.*

WHITE COOKIES.—One cup sugar, one-half cup butter, one egg beaten well, one-half cup sour milk, one half teaspoon soda, flavor with vanilla or nutmeg; flour enough to make a stiff batter. Let stand on ice for an hour, then roll out quickly, sift sugar on top and bake. All cookies are improved by keeping the dough as cold as possible.

MOLASSES SPONGE CAKE.—Yolks of two eggs, three tablespoons of sugar, slightly heaping; three-fourths cup molasses, one cup and three tablespoons flour. Ginger or not as you please. Mix all together thoroughly, then put three-fourths cup of boiling water, stir, then add teaspoon of soda wet in cold water.—*Mrs. C. J. Davis.*

SOFT GINGER CAKE.—One pound of lard, one quart molasses, quarter quart milk, two eggs, half ounce soda, one teaspoon ginger, flour enough to make it stiff.—*Mrs. F. Lutz.*

SOFT GINGER CAKE.—One-half cup of sour milk, one-half cup of sugar, one-half cup of molasses one-half cup of shortening (lard or drippings), one and one-half cups of flour, one egg and a little salt if lard is used; ginger and spices to taste, one teaspoon of soda. Beat egg, sugar and shortening well together, put soda into the molasses and stir in with the flour and other ingredients. Bake in a square tin one-half hour in a slow oven.—*Mrs. O. M. Barnes.*

GINGER CAKE.—One-half cup butter, one-half cup brown sugar, one cup New Orleans molasses, two cups unsifted Royal patent flour, stir together thoroughly, put one teaspoon soda and one teaspoon ginger in a cup and fill with boiling water, pour this into the dough, beat two eggs light and put these in last. Bake in a dripping pan or two bread tins. The batter will be quite thin but do not use any more flour.—*Mrs. C. F. Swift.*

DARK COOKIES.—One cup white sugar, one cup lard or (better) two-thirds cup cottolene, three eggs (beaten), one heaping teaspoon soda, one cup New Orleans molasses, one-fourth cup water, one small teaspoon salt, one even teaspoon cinnamon, one heaping teaspoon ginger, flour enough to mix soft.—*Mrs. Belle M. Perry, Charlotte.*

GINGER DROPS.—Half cup sugar, one cup molasses, half cup butter, two teaspoons soda in a cup boiling water, two and a half cups flour, add two well-beaten eggs, the last thing, cinnamon, ginger and salt to taste. —*Mrs. E. S. Porter.*

GINGER COOKIES.—One cup of molasses, one cup sugar, one full cup butter, one cup strong coffee, two teaspoons of soda, one teaspoon of ginger, one teaspoon of cinnamon, mix as soft as you can roll them out. —*Mrs. Crossman.*

MOLASSES COOKIES.—One and one-half cups of molasses, one-half cup of sugar, one cup of hot lard, two teaspoons of soda, little salt, ginger and cinnamon. Stir stiff with flour. Put this on the ice and let stand all night. Roll out in the morning and bake. By standing and getting ice cold they require less flour in rolling out and consequently are softer and richer than otherwise.—*Kittie Walker.*

DOUGHNUTS.

FRIED CAKES.—Beat two eggs with one cup of sugar, add a teacup of new milk, half a teaspoon of salt, sift two or three times one quart of flour and two heaping teaspoons of baking powder. Mix well together and fry in hot lard.—*Mrs. Johns.*

FRIED CAKES.—One and three-fourths cups C. sugar (light brown), three eggs, three large spoonfuls melted lard, cinnamon to taste, one cup sweet milk, two teaspoons baking powder, and flour to stiffen. Roll very soft.—*Mrs. J. J. Baird.*

EXCELLENT FRIED CAKES.—Seven tablespoons of granulated sugar, five tablespoons of melted butter, two eggs, nutmeg, seventeen tablespoons sweet milk, three heaping teaspoons Queen Flake baking powder, one quart Royal patent flour, measure flour before sifting, sift the baking powder with flour three times. Beat eggs and sugar well together, then add butter and milk. Mix soft.—*Mrs. Nellie R. Chapin.*

NO. 1 FRIED CAKES.—One cup sugar, one cup milk, three eggs, three scant tablespoons melted butter, three teaspoons baking powder, nutmeg, pinch of salt. Beat eggs well, add milk, sugar, butter, salt, nutmeg, baking powder and flour to make soft dough. Do not mix with hands till ready to roll out. Roll to thickness of a cracker and have lard almost smoking hot.—*Julia B. Judson.*

PICKLES AND SAUCES.

PEACH PICKLES.—Brush the peaches with a stiff brush, this will remove all the fuzz; then stick in each peach two Cassia buds and two cloves. To one bushel of peaches take twenty pounds of granulated sugar, one quart of vinegar. Boil this until sugar is dissolved, watching carefully and stirring gently so that it will not burn. Pick the peaches with silver fork and drop into syrup, few at a time, boil them and then skim out and put into a colander. After draining put into cans and pour hot syrup over them and seal hot. Do not crowd too many peaches into a can. Lay the cans on their side all night.

This recipe came from a large canning establishment in New York State and is most excellent.—*Ella W. Shank.*

FRENCH PICKLES.—One peck green tomatoes sliced, six large onions, one teacup salt. Mix these and let stand over night. Drain thoroughly and boil in one quart of vinegar mixed with two quarts of water for fifteen or twenty minutes, then drain.

Then take three quarts vinegar, two pounds brown sugar, two tablespoons of ground allspice, two tablespoons cinnamon, two tablespoons ginger, two tablespoons ground mustard. Moisten the mustard, then throw all together and boil fifteen minutes.—*Mrs. Lucy C. Davis.*

APPLE PICKLES.—Eleven pounds apples, three pounds sugar, two ounces cloves, two ounces cinnamon, one quart of good cider vinegar. Cook the apples until soft, then put the spiced vinegar on boiling hot.

PHILADELPHIA PICKLE.—One-half peck green tomatoes, one dozen large cucumbers, two large red peppers, one coffeecup of grated horseradish, two large onions, two small heads of cabbage, two ounces each of black and white mustard seed, two ounces of celery seed and half pint of salt. Chop onions, cabbage, cucumbers, tomatoes and peppers, add salt and let stand three hours, then drain dry; add one pound of sugar, put all together, mix thoroughly and add cider vinegar enough to cover. Will keep any length of time. Needs no cooking.—*Mary Bender.*

CHOWDER.—One gallon chopped green tomatoes, one gallon cabbage chopped fine, four onions, eight green peppers, chopped, two tablespoons of pepper, two tablespoons of cloves, three of cinnamon, three gills white mustard seed, one gill of salt, one pound of sugar, three quarts of vinegar, three tablespoons celery seed. Boil all together for an hour; stir well while cooking.—*Mrs. D. M. Hough.*

Mustard Pickles.—Two quarts cauliflower, two quarts small onions, two quarts cucumbers, two quarts green tomatoes, one-fourth dozen green peppers, soak in salt water twenty-four hours, drain and boil tender in weak vinegar, place in jar, take vinegar enough to cover pickels, three tablespoons of ground mustard, same of flour and one teaspoon of cinnamon with cold vinegar, mix with boiling vinegar and pour over pickles.—*Mrs. E. Perrin.*

Mustard Pickles.—Ten small heads of cauliflower, two quarts of small onions, eleven large cucumbers sliced into pieces about an inch thick, one-half gallon small cucumbers, one-half dozen green peppers sliced (seeds taken out), two quarts green tomatoes. These are all to lie in salt water twenty-four hours, then drain, boil in vinegar until tender, then boil two gallons of vinegar, mix one-half pound ground mustard, one-half pound flour into a little of the cold vinegar and when it begins to thicken add one tablespoon of turmeric and one pound brown sugar and pour over pickles. This is very nice, and if sealed in fruit cans will keep indefinitely.—*Mrs. Nancy Andrews.*

Pickled Cabbage.—Slice cabbages as fine as possible. For one head take one cup sugar, one teaspoonful of salt and one of pepper. Mix this together thoroughly and pack in crock over which pour scalding vinegar. This will keep all winter.

Pickled Raisins.—Leave two pounds raisins on the stems, add one pint vinegar, and one-half pound sugar. Simmer half an hour.—*Mrs. E. H. Whitney.*

Chili Sauce.—Two dozen large tomatoes, three onions, one green pepper, three teaspoons ground cinnamon, one of cloves, one of allspice, one and one-half cup brown sugar, two cups vinegar. Boil till quite thick, add the vinegar just before bottling.—*Mrs. M. W. Howard.*

Tomato Catsup.—Cook and strain through a course sieve to remove the seeds and skins, then add to each gallon when cold four tablespoons of salt level full, three tablespoons of ground mustard, two tablespoons of black pepper, one tablespoon of ground allspice, one-half tablespoon of cloves, a little bit of red pepper and a pint of vinegar. Simmer slowly four hours.—*Mrs. Barton.*

Spiced Currants.—Five pounds currants, four pounds of sugar, one pint of vinegar, four teaspoons of each of cinnamon and cloves. Boil three hours.

Cucumber Catsup.—Take two quarts of green cucumbers chopped fine, let them drain twelve hours, then add a large cup of onions, also chopped fine, one-half cup salt, one-half cup molasses, one tablespoon of pepper, just enough vinegar to cover. Put in bottles or small cans for future use.—*Fannie L. Chaffee.*

Tomato Butter.—Seven pounds of ripe tomatoes (pared), three pounds of sugar, one ounce cinnamon, ground, one-half ounce cloves, ground, one pint good cider vinegar. Boil three hours. Will keep without sealing.—*Mary R. Bryant.*

Cold Tomato Catsup.—One peck of ripe tomatoes, pare and chop fine; drain well to get all the water from them, then put three pints of good cider vinegar over them and let stand while preparing the following: One and one-half cups of chopped onions, two cups sugar, one cup grated horse-radish, one-half pound white mustard seed, two teaspoonfuls black pepper, four even teaspoonfuls cinnamon, one teaspoon of cloves, one teaspoon of mace (if liked), two large red peppers, chopped, two cups of chopped celery, mix all with tomatoes and vinegar. Put in fruit cans or seal in bottles.—*Mrs. F. F. Reymick, Saginaw.*

Grape Catsup.—Let five pints grapes simmer till soft enough to rub, all but the seeds through a colander. Then add two pints brown sugar, one pint vinegar, two tablespoons allspice, two tablespoons cloves, two tablespoons cinnamon, one and one-half teaspoons mace, one teaspoon salt, one-half teaspoon red pepper. Boil slowly till thick enough.—*Mrs. E. H. Whitney.*

Spiced Cherries.—Two quarts pitted cherries, one cup of raisins (chopped), two lemons (juice and chopped rind), three pints sugar, one tablespoon cinnamon, one-half tablespoon cloves. Boil all together one hour, or till thick.—*Mrs. C. J. Davis.*

Mustard Catsup.—One peck of tomatoes, stew half an hour; then add one-half cup of salt, two teaspoons black pepper, one-half ounce mace flakes, two teacups of chopped onions, one cup of brown sugar, boil half an hour, then strain; then add one-half pound mustard mixed with one pint of vinegar, just let come to a boil and seal up in bottles.—*Mrs. Chas. Shubel.*

Salad Dressing for Eggs.—Yolk of one egg, one small teaspoon of salt, one-half of pepper, one of mustard, one large spoon of sugar, one tablespoon of butter, four of vinegar, four of sweet milk, if too thick when cold, thin with sweet cream.

Meat Sauce.—One dozen green tomatoes, one dozen ripe tomatoes, six onions, four large apples, one red pepper, one pound raisins, one pound sugar, one tablespoonful each of cloves, cinnamon and allspice; add one quart of vinegar.—*Mrs. H. P. Bartlett.*

CANDY.

"All the labor of man is for his mouth,
And yet the appetite is not filled."

French Cream.—Whites of two eggs and half as much water; add flavoring and stir them together well, but do not beat, then mix in two pounds confectioner's sugar.

Nut Creams—Chop almonds, butternuts, hickorynuts or English walnuts quite fine; make "French Cream" and before adding all the sugar. While cream is soft stir in nuts, form into balls, cubes or bars.

Molasses Candy.—Two cups molasses, one cup of sugar, one tablespoon of vinegar, butter size of a hickorynut, boil until it will make a hard wax, when ready to take off add a teaspoon of soda and stir briskly, pull and cut with scissors.

Maple Praulien.—Take one cup maple sugar, add a very little water and boil until it strings, then add one-half cupful hickory nuts shelled and broken in small pieces, then put into buttered pans to cool.

Lemon Drops.—Pour clear lemon juice upon powdered sugar and boil until a thick syrup; drop upon plates singly and dry in a warm place.

Pop Corn Balls.—Six quarts popped corn; boil two cups of sugar, butter size of an egg, one-quarter cup of vinegar; one-quarter cup of water, until it is brittle dropped in cold water; stir this quickly into the corn, cover, dip hands into cold water and mold into balls while hot.

CREAM PEPPERMINTS.—One pint granulated sugar, six tablespoons hot water, boil together four minutes. Take from stove and add twelve drops essence of peppermint, one-half teaspoon of cream of tartar, and one tablespoon of powdered sugar. Beat this mixture exactly two minutes and drop with spoon on paper quickly and they will harden.

PEANUT CANDY.—Two cups granulated sugar, one cup chopped peanuts; put sugar in iron spider without water, stir constantly until melted, being careful not to burn, when melted stir in peanuts quickly and pour into unbuttered pans to cool.—*Anna Brackett.*

VASSAR GIRLS' FUDGE.—Two teacups granulated sugar, one teacup sweet milk, piece of butter size of walnut, teaspoon vanilla, pinch salt, one square Baker's chocolate. Put in stew pan and cook till it hardens in water. Take from stove and stir hard for two or three minutes. Pour on buttered tin and mark off in squares.—*Mrs. B. F. Hall.*

HOME-MADE FRENCH CANDY.—The unbeaten white of one egg, to this add powdered sugar which has been rolled smooth, stir till thick, dropping the flavoring in a drop at a time, then knead with the fingers till it has the appearance of a ball of pie dough, then mould in balls about as large as a hickory nut. Press this against the side of a cut glass dish to make fancy candies, or press halves of English walnuts on them, or with a hat pin dip into chocolate as prepared for cake frosting, lay on greased paper. They are ready for use the next day after making. To make pink candies put one tablespoonful of red sugar in the egg before adding powdered sugar.—*Mrs. C. C. Wood.*

MAPLE SUGAR CANDY.—One cup sweet cream, two cups maple sugar, broken fine. Let it boil slowly and do not stir more than necessary. When it thickens in cold water, pour in buttered tins and cut in squares.

CREAM CANDY.—One half cup sweet milk, with a little vanilla to flavor. When it boils add two cups sugar and let it boil hard five minutes, stiring it constantly. Then remove from fire and stir thoroughly until cold. When it becomes thick, spread upon buttered plates.—*Mrs. G. H. House.*

Chocolate and White Layer Candy.—Cover two cups of sugar with water and boil till it strings a little, then pour half of the mixture into another dish and add a square of chocolate, melted, and one teaspoon of vanilla. Stir both until fine grained, then put on a buttered plate, first a layer of white and then a layer of chocolate mixture, and so on.—*Elizabeth O' Connor.*

MISCELLANEOUS.

"It is safe to say that the food wasted in American homes, if utilized, would abundantly feed our hungry poor. We have never sufficiently considered the part which the wise economy of the housekeeper plays in creating wealth."

Bancroft House Hash.—Corned beef and boiled potatoes, cold when chopped and not chopped too fine. Use one cup of meat, three cups of potatoes, one-fourth cup of butter, one half cup of milk. Stew in saucepan over a slow fire and serve plain or browned in a frying pan, omelet shape.—*Farnham Lyon.*

Baked Hash.—Hash veal, corned or roasted beef, or any meat or combination of meats, season with pepper and salt. Wet with chicken broth or any soup stock, or with cream or milk. To this add mashed potato beaten with the white of an egg, two teaspoons of cream, salt and pepper. Put all into a well-greased baking pan; bake half or three-quarters of an hour. Use equal parts of potato and meat. When done turn upon a platter and serve.

Oysters in Chafing Dish.—Put in chafing dish two tablespoons of butter, one saltspoon of salt and same of pepper. Drain the oysters from the liquor and add to the other ingredients. When cooked, pour over heated crackers.—*Saginaw Cook Book.*

A Chafing Dish Dainty.—Here is a delicious and simple chafing dish dainty. Split some crackers, butter both halves generously, sprinkle over a rich layer of cheese, set in chafing dish and dust lightly with cayenne; cover and place the dish over spirit lamp until the cheese melts.—*Saginaw Cook Book.*

NUTS AND RAISINS.—The place of these in the bill of fare has been made at the end, and as both are substantial food they have at the end of a heavy meal been the one thing too much and so been set down as indigestible. Brain workers a good while ago found that a bunch of raisins with light crackers or a slice of bread made not only a satisfactory lunch, but one on which they could work easily, and in many cases nuts have taken the place of bread, though they go well together, a sandwich of thin, lightly buttered bread and English walnuts being particularly good. The oil of the richer nuts is especially nourishing, but every variety requires long and very thorough chewing. Eaten in this way with raisins they form one of the best possible foods, and their value is just being recognized by the physician who studies dietaries.—*Helen Campbell.*

STUFFED DATES.—Take a pound of dates and remove the pits and replace them with pecan meats. Fold them over and mould them into ovals and roll them in pulverized sugar.—*Miss Alice Daily.*

GRAPE JUICE.—Take ten pounds of grapes, two quarts of water and let simmer until soft enough to press out the juice, then return to the stove, add two cups sugar, let boil, skim and bottle hot. Use Concord prapes.—*Mrs. George H. House.*

LEMONADE.—The juice of eight lemons and of four oranges, sweeten to taste and add two quarts of cold water and two well-beaten fresh eggs, add shaved ice and mix all together.—*Miss Daily.*

RASPBERRY SHRUB.—Place red raspberries in a stone jar, cover them with good cider vinegar, let stand over night, next morning strain and to one pint of juice add one pint of sugar, boil ten minutes, bottle while hot.—*Charlotte Cook Book.*

CURRANT SHRUB.—To three pints of strained currant juice add one pound of white sugar, boil fifteen minutes, skim it well, when cool bottle and cork. This is used with ice water as a drink.—*Charlotte Cook Book.*

COFFEE.—For two hundred people take five pounds coffee, five eggs, a little salt; mix in cold water, place in bags, put in the boiler and steep, not boil.—*Mrs. John Jones.*

GINGERED PEARS.—Four pounds pears chopped fine, four pounds sugar, one ounce green ginger root chopped fine, grated rind of four lemons; make syrup of one pint water and sugar, add fruit, ginger root, and lemon rind, cook until clear, put in tumblers or jars.—*Miss Cornelia Sibbald, Saginaw.*

TO COOK CRANBERRIES.—Have one pint of water *boiling* in a porcelain or granite kettle. To this add two quarts of cranberries and cover closely. As soon as the fruit boils thoroughly add a small pinch of soda, and stir lightly, cover and boil five minutes or until the berries are well broken, then add two cups of granulated sugar, more or less according to taste. Simmer on top of stove for five or ten minutes. Turn into earthen dish to cool. Tin spoils both color and flavor. Always have water *boiling*, otherwise the fruit becomes tough and bitter.—*Mrs. N. B. Jones.*

QUINCE HONEY.—Two cups grated quince, two cups water, four cups sugar. Boil until thick.—*Mrs. W. E. Trager.*

USEFUL HINTS.

The following is a list of articles prepared for the entertainment of 300 persons by a Boston caterer, who uses turkeys for salads as being cheaper than chickens, as there is more meat in proportion to the bone: Fifty pounds turkey, two hams, four tongues, one dozen bunehes celery, six bottles sweet oil, six quarts cream, four dozen eggs, ten gallons oysters, prepared with powdered crackers, six pounds coffee, seventy pounds of wedding cake, forty of bride, sponge and angel cakes, fancy cakes and confectionery at pleasure.—*Mrs. M. W. Howard.*

STAINS AND THEIR REMOVAL.—For the removal of stains and spots from colored materials and carpets, ammonia takes the first place. Almost any mark, new or old, will yield to its perservering use, and if dabbed on (not rubbed) it will itself leave no trace of its use. It can be applied to woolens, cottons and silk. It will remove ink spots from marble, paper and wood; and when diluted with water, spots caused by orange or lemon juice are removed by it from the most delicate materials. From carpets and curtains and suits of clothing it will remove almost every stain, including that caused by whitewash. Benzine will remove paint from delicate fabrics; if it fails, turpentine must be used, and the mark which it leaves effaced by alcohol. If in the process of removing stains the color departs from the material, it can generally be restored by dabbing with chloroform.—*Mrs. D. M. Hough.*

Here is a receipt that will knock out the carpet bug every time. One ounce of alum, one ounce of chloride of zinc, and three ounces of salt. Mix with one quart of water and let it stand over night in a covered vessel, so that all sediment may be left behind. Dilute this with two quarts of water and apply by sprinkling the edges of the carpet about a foot from the wall. This is all that is necessary. They will leave boxes, bedding and any other resort which has been sprinkled with the solution, on the shortest possible notice, and nothing will be injured in texture or color.—*Mrs. Wm. Donovan, Mrs. N. B. Jones.*

"Saving is a more difficult art than earning."

"The real science of cooking is to be able to cook a good meal or dish with but little out of which to make it."

"If you attempt the boiling to hurry, the wood only is wasted;
But in attempting the baking to hurry, the food as well isn't fit to be tasted."

The words of the late Prof. Blot, founder of the New York Cooking Academy, in his advice to cooks, were: "Be careful, clean and punctual. Make use of everything good and waste nothing, however little it may be. Have no prejudices."

Two apples kept in the cake box and renewed when shriveled will keep the cake moist.

A pinch of powdered sugar and another of cornstarch beaten in with the yolks of eggs will keep an omelet from collapsing. Beat the whites stiff and then cut them into the yolks.

If ham is very salt freshen by placing in cold water one hour before cooking. Never use tepid or hot water as it toughens the meat.

In lemon pies, vinegar may be substituted for lemons, or one lemon used for flavoring and the remainder vinegar.

Set a dish filled with water in the oven with baking bread or cake and it will seldom scorch.

To keep a little "left over" pie dough till the next baking, grease it all over with lard and set in a cool place.—*Mrs. C. C. Wood.*

To remove ink spots from linen or cotton dip the spots in pure melted tallow, then wash out the tallow and the ink will invariably come with it.

"Water in boiling loses the air or gases which give it a fresh taste and sparkling appearance, it becomes flat and tasteless, therefore it is very important in making tea and coffee to have it freshly boiled."

"Fresh water boils at two hundred twelve degrees; salt water at two hundred twenty-four degrees. If we salt the water in the lower part of the double boiler a greater degree of heat is obtained by which to cook the articles in the top."

If any food be spilled upon the stove while cooking, immediately throw salt upon it and there will be no disagreeable smell arising from it.—*Mrs. Edward Talbort.*

A few bread crumbs tied up in a bag and thrown into a kettle of boiling cabbage will effectually destroy the unpleasant odor.—*Mrs. Edward Talbort.*

COUGH SYRUP.—Recommended as a constitutional remedy where there is low vitality and an obstinate cough, especially good in cases of cough following la grippe One ounce each of skunk cabbage root, wild turnip root, sarsaparilla root, golden seal and white root, one-half ounce blood root, one-fourth ounce mandrake root, three ounces white resin. Put all except the last in a thin muslin bag and boil in one quart of water until reduced to one pint. Then remove the bag of roots, squeeze dry as possible, and add resin pulverized, and one pound of loaf sugar. Simmer half an hour. When nearly cold add two tablespoonfuls of alcohol and bottle. Dose for adult, one teaspoonful three times a day.—*Mrs. N. B. Jones.*

FOR A COUGH —One-half cup of flax seed, two quarts of water, boil one hour, strain through a thin cloth and add half a teacup of sugar and the juice of three lemons.—*Mrs. John Whiteley.*

CURE FOR THE HURT OF A RUSTY NAIL.—Apply to the parts a bran mash made with weak lye and change often —*C. M. C.*

HOP BITTERS.—Two ounces hops, one-half ounce buchu, one-half ounce extract of dandelion, one-half pint of alcohol, one-half pound of sugar, twenty drops of mandrake. Boil the hops and buchu together one hour, then add the rest of the ingredients. This is a splendid tonic for the spring of the year.

UNFERMENTED WINE.—To ten pounds of Concord grapes take four pounds of granulated sugar, wash the fruit and remove from the stems and let them boil twenty minutes, then strain and boil twenty minutes and add the sugar, sealing it while hot. This is delicious in case of sickness.

Try lime water for chilblains, one-half pound of stone lime to one pint of water, let settle and strain. Apply at bed time.

For a severe burn slice turnips into unsalted boiling lard, and cook slowly until thoroughly crisped. Strain carefully and apply lard as ointment. Will heal and prevent scarring when other remedies fail to relieve.—*Mrs. Marcia Jones.*

For a cough steep one cup crushed sunflower seeds and one cup of sugar with sufficient water to melt sugar, simmer slowly for an hour. Strain and give in teaspoonful doses as often as necessary to control cough.

PERMANGANATE OF POTASH AS A DISINFECTANT.—There's nothing so magical in its cleansing results as permanganate of potash. A few crystals dissolved in a pail of warm water will sweeten a musty cupboard, and will freshen all disagreeable-smelling articles to which water can be applied. Five cents worth dissolved in a quart of water and added, a little at a time, to a cistern of ill-smelling water will remove all offensive odor.

Table of Contents.

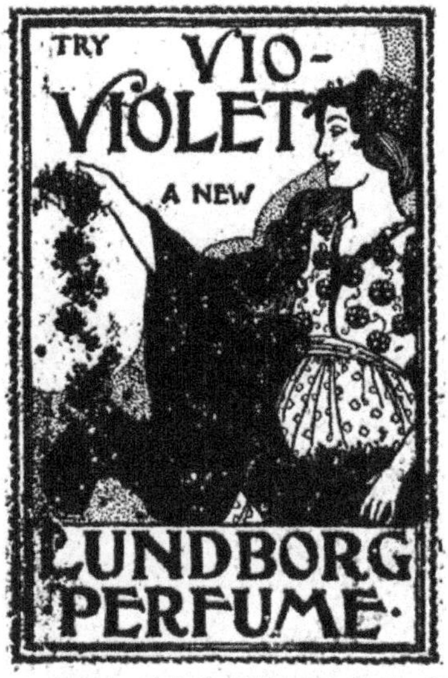
TRY
VIO-
VIOLET
A NEW
LUNDBORG
PERFUME

Made in the USA
Monee, IL
04 November 2026

67378956R00075